Lecture Notes in Computer Science 2230

Edited by G. Goos, J. Hartmanis, and J. van Leeuwen

W0231993

Springer
Berlin
Heidelberg
New York
Barcelona
Hong Kong
London
Milan
Paris
Tokyo

Toivo Katila   Isabelle E. Magnin
Patrick Clarysse   Johan Montagnat
Jukka Nenonen (Eds.)

Functional Imaging and Modeling of the Heart

First International Workshop, FIMH 2001
Helsinki, Finland, November 15-16, 2001
Proceedings

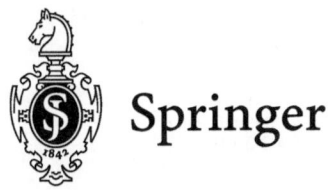 Springer

Series Editors

Gerhard Goos, Karlsruhe University, Germany
Juris Hartmanis, Cornell University, NY, USA
Jan van Leeuwen, Utrecht University, The Netherlands

Volume Editors

Toivo Katila
Jukka Nenonen
Helsinki University of Technology, Institute of Biomedical Engineering
P.O. Box 2200, 02015 Finland
E-mail: {Toivo.Katila,Jukka.Nenonen}@hut.fi

Isabelle E. Magnin
Patrick Clarysse
Johan Montagnat
CREATIS, CNRS, INSA, bâtiment Blaise Pascal
20, boulevard Albert Einstein, 69621 Villeurbanne cedex, France
E-mail: {Isabelle.Magnin,Patrick.Clarysse,Johan.Montagnat}@creatis.insa-lyon.fr

Cataloging-in-Publication Data applied for

Die Deutsche Bibliothek - CIP-Einheitsaufnahme

Functional imaging and modeling of the heart : first international workshop ;
proceedings / FIMH 2001, Helsinki, Finland, November 15 - 16, 2001.
Toivo Katila ... (ed.). - Berlin ; Heidelberg ; New York ; Barcelona ; Hong Kong ;
London ; Milan ; Paris ; Tokyo : Springer, 2002
    (Lecture notes in computer science ; Vol. 2230)
    ISBN 3-540-42861-5

CR Subject Classification (1998): I.4, J.3, I.6, I.2.10

ISSN 0302-9743
ISBN 3-540-42861-5 Springer-Verlag Berlin Heidelberg New York

Springer-Verlag Berlin Heidelberg New York
a member of BertelsmannSpringer Science+Business Media GmbH

http://www.springer.de

© Springer-Verlag Berlin Heidelberg 2001

Typesetting: Camera-ready by author, data conversion by PTP-Berlin, Stefan Sossna
Printed on acid-free paper   SPIN: 10845753   06/3142   5 4 3 2 1 0

Preface

The recent developments in dynamic cardiac imaging and modeling are the result of an increasingly fruitful cooperation between theoreticians, engineers, and practitioners. The standard clinical parameters are progressively benefitting from more accurate quantitative measurements thanks to a simultaneous use of sophisticated data acquisition techniques such as multichannel ECG and MEG, dynamic US, doppler, X-Ray, CT, helical CT, MRI, fMRI, SPECT, PET... data and advanced physical and mathematical tools. It is becoming possible to efficiently combine prior anatomical and functional knowledge with advanced 3D spatio-temporal digital data. The challenge now is clearly to correlate the micro structure and function of the organ from the cellular level with its macroscopic functional behavior.

The FIMH 2001 international workshop aimed to promote collaboration between scientists in signal and image processing, applied mathematics and physics, biomedical engineering and computer science, and experts in cardiology, radiology, biology, and physiology. The FIMH 2001 workshop, in its first year, focused on complex heart models involving anatomical and functional information. The goal is to gradually move toward hybrid 3D biomechanical and electrophysiological models able to simulate the dynamic behavior of the heart.

We feel that FIMH 2001 presented an opportunity to create a cardio-vascular research network at a European level to federate the main pluridisciplinary groups involved in advanced research in cardiovascular imaging and modeling in Europe. The idea is to create what could be called the "European Beating Heart Project". The purpose of such a project is to join research efforts to improve diagnosis and therapy of pathological dysfunctions of the heart, for the benefit of the patient, through fundamental and clinical research.

September 2001   Toivo Katila
                                                           Isabelle E. Magnin

Acknowledgements

The members of the program committee deserve special thanks for their job in reviewing all the papers, and for their support in the organization of the conference.

We thank the members of the CREATIS unit in Lyon and the Laboratory of Biomedical Engineering in Helsinki for their involvement and support in the organization of this conference.

Conference supported by

Institut National des Sciences Appliquées de Lyon (INSA), France
Helsinki University of Technology (HUT), Finland
Centre National de la Recherche Scientifique (CNRS), France
Science Academy of Finland
Joint incentive action "Beating Heart" of the CNRS, France
French Cultural Center, Helsinki
French-Finnish Association for Scientific and Technical Research (AFFRST)
French Biomedical Engineering Society (SFGBM)

Organization

FIMH 2001 was co-organized by the CREATIS Laboratory, CNRS UMR 5515, Lyon, France, and the Laboratory of Biomedical Engineering at the Helsinski University of Technology, Finland.

Conference Chairs

Toivo Katila   Laboratory of Biomedical Engineering, Helsinski University of Technology, Finland
Isabelle E. Magnin   CREATIS, CNRS UMR 5515, Lyon, France

Organization Committee

Patrick Clarysse   CREATIS, CNRS UMR 5515, Lyon, France
Johan Montagnat   CREATIS, CNRS UMR 5515, Lyon, France
Jukka Nenonen   Laboratory of Biomedical Engineering, Helsinski University of Technology, Finland

Program Committee

T. Arts   University of Technology of Eindhoven, The Netherlands
N. Ayache   INRIA Sophia-Antipolis, France
S. Baillet   La Pitié Salpétrière, Paris, France
M. Barlaud   I3S, Sophia-Antipolis, France
L. Bidaut   Hôpitaux Universitaires de Genève, Switzerland
B. Bijnens   MIC, Katholieke Universiteit Leuven, Belgium
I. Bloch   ENST, Paris, France
E. Canet   CREATIS, Lyon, France
P. Clarysse   CREATIS, Lyon, France
L. Cohen   CEREMADE, Paris, France
P. Croisille   CREATIS, Lyon, France
J. Declerck   OMIA, Oxford, United Kingdom
H. Delingette   INRIA Sophia-Antipolis, France
J. D'hooge   MIC, Katholieke Universiteit Leuven, Belgium
R. Fenici   Catholic University of Rome, Italy
D. Friboulet   CREATIS, Lyon, France
A. Herment   INSERM U494, Paris, France
M. Horacek   Dalhousie University, Canada
M. Janier   CREATIS, Lyon, France
H. Larson   Hvidovre Hospital, Denmark
K. Lauerma   Helsinki University Central Hospital, Finland

Program Committee (continuation)

S. Loncaric	University of Zagreb, Croatia
J. Lötjönen	VTT Technology, Tampere, Finland
I. E. Magnin	CREATIS, Lyon, France
M. Mäkijärvi	Helsinki University Central Hospital, Helsinki, Finland
J. Meunier	Université de Montréal, Canada
J. Montagnat	CREATIS, Lyon, France
P. Nekkola	University of Technology, Munich, Germany
J. Nenonen	Helsinki University of Technology, Finland
A. Noble	Medical Vision Laboratory, Oxford, United Kingdom
J. Ohayon	Université de Savoie, France
M. Orkisz	CREATIS, Lyon, France
N. Rougon	ARTEMIS, Institut National des Télécommunication d'Evry, France
C. Roux	ENST Bretagne, France
P. Rubel	INSERM U121, Lyon, France
F. Sachse	University of Karlsruhe, Germany
J. Sequeira	LIM, Marseille, France
G. Sutherland	MIC, Katholieke Universiteit Leuven, Belgium
B. Tilg	University of Graz, Austria
Y. Usson	TIMC, Grenoble, France
Y.-M. Zhu	CREATIS, Lyon, France

Table of Contents

Modules in Cardiac Modeling: Mechanics, Circulation, and Depolarization Wave

T. Arts[1,2], P. Bovendeerd[2], A. van der Toorn[1], L. Geerts[2], R. Kerckhoffs[1,2], and F. Prinzen[3].

Department of Biophysics[1] and Physiology[3],
Maastricht University, Maastricht, The Netherlands.
[2]Faculty of Biomedical Engineering, Technological University Eindhoven,
Eindhoven, The Netherlands
t.arts@bf.unimaas.nl

Abstract. Numerical models of various aspects of cardiac function are useful in simulating pathologies and therapies. Such models cannot be easily combined because of differences in input and output structure. To harbor the different models we have developed a framework, consisting of a graph network with nodes (compliant cavities) and edges (flow ducts). Thus using a toolkit of modules facilitates tailored cardiac modeling.

1 Introduction

Numerical models of cardiac mechanics are expected to be valuable tools in simulating cardiac pathologies and evaluating different strategies for therapy. In designing a cardiac simulation, one has to decide, which physiological mechanisms have to be included in a simulation. Important aspects may be modification of the depolarization wave by the degree of stretch of the myocardial tissue, coronary flow dynamics, the metabolic supply-demand balance of the myocardial tissue, the internal fiber structure within the heart, and adaptation of the structure to changes in load.

In modeling cardiac function in more detail, interaction with the rest of the circulation is crucial. Focussing on the heart, a cardiac beat is initiated by a depolarization wave originating in sinus node, spreading out subsequently over the atria, the atrioventricular node, and both ventricles. As a consequence the heart contracts. Pressure rises in the ventricles. After exceeding pressure in the large arteries the outflow valves open. While the myocardium relaxes, flow diminishes and the outflow valves close. Then, the pressure head from the atria to the ventricular cavities causes the atrioventricular valve to open, resulting in filling.

If regional myocardial function is a focus, the circulation is an important boundary condition to the mechanics of the wall. Venous pressures determine diastolic filling. Arterial pressures determine outflow phenomena. The balance of inflow and outflow determines the volumes in the cardiac cavities. When knowing the latter volumes, numerical models of cardiac mechanics may be used to determine global and local mechanical load of the myocardium as a function of time.

Currently, most models of cardiac mechanics are focussed on one cavity, generally the left ventricle. Boundary conditions, set by the circulation to cavity mechanics, are

T. Katila et al. (Eds.): FIMH 2001, LNCS 2230, pp. 1-9, 2001.

often simplified to a preload and afterload pressure level. One may think of simulating the mechanics of the various cavities with their mutual interactions during for instance pacing. These interactions are very sensitive to relative timing of events in the various cavities, thus needing to include the circulation in the model.

Because most models are made with a specific goal, little attention has been paid on combining the strength of the various models. They are generally not suited to be mutually combined. On may solve this problem by simulating all cardiac and circulatory mechanisms in great detail and as accurate as possible according to current physiological knowledge. Despite optimism about increasing possibilities in computing, such approach is not likely to work. According to standard rules in modeling strategy, one should first determine the goal of the simulation. In reducing modeling efforts to a minimum a focus is chosen near which accuracy should be as high as required. Further from the focus accuracy may be less, thus enabling important savings of effort. A disadvantage of this approach is that each problem will result in a different model, generally not compatible with other models.

The question arises how to combine the advantages of one comprehensive and accurate model with the tailored and much faster models. We propose to think in modules. The framework of the circulation model should be a working, simple and well-structured model of the circulation with the heart. When choosing a focus of simulation, more accurate ones should replace modules near the focus. When replacing a module, the structure of communication with the rest of the model should be left unaffected. Ideally, a toolkit of modules with standard interfacings should be available. For a specific problem, the appropriate tools should be selected and composed to a tailored, complete model system. An important advantage of this approach is that developed specific modules can be used in other applications and by other groups so that not much modeling work has to be repeated.

In the present study we introduce a working model of the circulation, having a modular structure, and containing a very limited number of module types. The structure is that of a mathematical graph, containing nodes interconnected with edges. The nodes are compliant cavities, and the edges are flow ducts with inertia and resistance. A cardiac chamber module is a non-linear time dependent compliant cavity. A valve is a non-linear, flow-direction sensitive resistance with inertia. For each module the type is defined, the list of parameters required by the type function, and the interconnection with the other modules. Thus a lumped model of circulatory dynamics is obtained, leading to a set of differential equations. Cavities and ducts have as state variable volume and flow, respectively. The derivatives of the related state variables follow from the module functions.

A few examples will be shown of focussing by replacing modules by more accurate ones, leaving the basic structure of the model intact. The examples concern the introduction of 1) sarcomere fiber dynamics, 2) transmural gradients in myofiber mechanics, and 3) finite element analysis of electrophysiological depolarization wave and ventricular mechanics.

2 Setup of the Model

The model of the circulation contains cavities as nodes, interconnected with flow ducts as edges, thus forming a graph network. The definition of the model is transformed to a system of differential equations in a set of state variables. State variables are linked to cavities and ducts. Knowing the values of all state variables, the state of the system is fully determined. Solution of the system of equations requires that 1) the derivatives of the state variables are expressed as a function of the state variables themselves, and 2) the values of all state variables are known at the starting moment of the simulation.

2.1 The Module of Type Cavity

A node of the model represents a cavity V. Pressure p in this cavity is a function of its volume:

$$p = \text{function}(V) \tag{1}$$

Most collagen based passive elastic biological cavities may be modeled by an exponential pressure volume relationship (7). In the circulatory system many cavities contain muscular tissues in the wall, among of which the cardiac chambers are the most obvious ones. The pressure p in such a chamber depends on cavity volume V and time t. The simplest model is a conventional passive elastic chamber, completed with a variable elastance model (8, 9):

$$p = p_{pass}\left(e^{(V-V_{pass,0})/V_{pass}} - 1\right) + E_{max}(t)(V - V_{act,0}) \tag{2}$$

Parameters p_{pas}, $V_{pass,0}$ and V_{pass} are linked to the passive element. Parameter $V_{act,0}$ represents the small residual volume, at which no active pressure can be developed. The function $E_{max}(t)$ contains the time function of activation. The moment t=0 defines initiation of the contraction cycle.

For the solution of the differential equation the time derivative of the cavity volume is expressed as the sum of flows q_i in the ducts directed to the cavity:

$$\frac{dV}{dt} = \sum_i q_i \tag{3}$$

2.2 The Module of Type Duct

An edge of the model represents a duct having inertia and resistance. Flow is a state variable. In modeling the duct, the time derivative of flow must be calculated as a function of flow and pressures in the proximal (p_{prox}) and distal node (p_{dist}). It holds:

$$\frac{dq}{dt} = \text{function}(p_{prox}, p_{dist}, q) \tag{4}$$

The pressures are a function of the volumes in the nodes by the pressure volume relation according to Eq. (1-2). Thus, for a duct the important condition is satisfied that the derivative of the state variable q is a function of state variables. Consider a duct as an inertia in series with a resistive module. The pressure drop p_r over the non-linear resistive component is a function of flow q:

$$p_r = \text{function}(q) \tag{5}$$

If this function is linear, the resistive part of the flow duct is a linear resistance. The remaining pressure over the inertia is the pressure drop $p_{prox} - p_{dist}$ over the duct minus the resistive pressure drop p_r. The inertia may be non-linear. For the flow derivative it holds:

$$\frac{dq}{dt} = \text{function}(p_{prox} - p_{dist} - p_r, q) \tag{6}$$

Note that a bloodvessel segment may be modeled by a cascade of compliant cavities alternated with inertive ducts. Such model simulates realistic conduction properties of the arterial pulse wave.

We have modeled a cardiac valve as a duct with inertia in series with a non-linear resistance. The physical background of the resistive part has been modeled as flow through an orifice with area A, which depends on current flow and on pressure drop. Furthermore, there may be a resistance R in series with the valve. The valve is considered open if either flow or pressure drop or both are positive. Thus Eq. (5) is specified to:

$$p_r = \frac{\rho\, q \cdot |q|}{2A^2} + qR \quad \text{with} \quad A = \begin{cases} (q > 0) \cup (p_{prox} > p_{dist}) & : A_{open} \\ \text{else} & : A_{leak} \end{cases} \tag{7}$$

Note that A_{leak} may be negligibly small, but not zero. The time derivative of flow is determined by the remaining pressure loss over the inertia, modeled by a flow channel with length l and area A. Thus Eq. (6) is specified to:

$$\frac{dq}{dt} = \frac{A(p_{prox} - p_{dist} - p_r)}{\rho l} \tag{8}$$

Parameters ρ, R, A_{open}, A_{leak}, and l are parameters to be provided.

If a duct is a resistance without inertia, flow itself is not a state variable in the set of differential equations, but it is a straightforward function of the state variables of the proximal and distal cavities:

$$q = (p_{prox} - p_{dist})/R_{duct} \tag{9}$$

2.3 Implementation

The structure of cavities interconnected with ducts is convenient as long as cavity volumes are state variables. It is inconvenient to have nodes not having volume as a state variable because then duct flows become mutually inconveniently coupled. To circumvent such problems it may useful to attribute some compliance to the cavity. The related time constants in the differential equation should be kept sufficiently small to keep phase errors negligible and sufficiently large to maintain numerical stability.

When setting up the simulation, it is important to decide what minimum rise time will be allowed for the dynamical behavior. For numerical stability all modules should have time constants not shorter than this rise time.

2.4 Design of the Circulation Model

The dynamic model of the normal circulation contains a systemic and a pulmonary tract (fig 1). Ducts interconnect cavities. This model will be used as the basic structure of cardiovascular modeling. Specific features can be focussed on by replacing modules by more detailed ones, while maintaining the original links. New ducts can be added to simulate many types of shunts, such as fistulas and cardiac shunts in newborns.

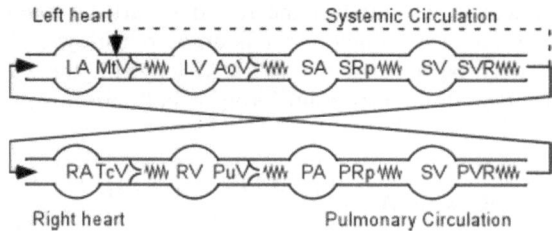

Fig. 1. The circulation has been modeled by a left and a right circuit of compliant cavities, interconnected by ducts, such as valves and resistances. The dashed arrow indicates a shortcut, used when focussing on simulating left ventricular hemodynamics. Then the LV module was replaced by a more accurate one.3 Specific Simulations

3 Specific Simulations

The model setup has been used to simulate the boundary conditions set to models, focussing on cardiac mechanics. As examples we have chosen 1) replacing the variable elastance model by a first order stress-strain model of the sarcomere, and coupling of sarcomere dynamics to left ventricular cavity mechanics, 2) relating cardiac deformation as measured with MRI with regional myofiber mechanics, 3) the effects of changing the pacing site on the ventricle for the sequence of local myofiber contraction.

3.1 Linking Ventricular Dynamics to Sarcomere Dynamics

In the model of Fig. 1, pressure of the left ventricle is calculated from its volume by an equation of type Eq. (1). In linking ventricular dynamics to sarcomere dynamics, local differences are considered not to exist. So we used a simple 1-fiber model as presented earlier (1). The strength of this model is its accurate description of the non-linear relationships between cavity volume V_{cav} and pressure p_{cav} on the one hand, and sarcomere length l_s and myofiber stress s_f on the other. It holds by good approximation:

$$l_s = l_{s0}\left(1+3\frac{V_{cav}}{V_{wall}}\right)^{1/3} \quad \text{and} \quad p_{cav} = \left(1+3\frac{V_{cav}}{V_{wall}}\right)s_f\left(l_s,t\right) \tag{10}$$

Parameter V_{wall} represents wall volume and l_{s0} is a scaling length for sarcomere length in the wall. In maintaining the links with the circulation model, Eq. (10) is used to express pressure p_{cav} as a function of cavity volume V_{cav}, given that the expression $s_f(l_s,t)$ for myofiber stress is known. For the latter expression we have used a first order Maxwell model, consisting of a passive elastic element in parallel with a series combination of a contractile element with length l_{CE} and a series elastic element l_{SE}. Velocity of contraction dl_{CE}/dt for the contractile element depends on external load and on the degree of activation, incorporated in the function $s_{iso}(t)$. We have used:

$$s_{pass} = s_{pass0}\left(e^{k(l_s-l_{s0})}-1\right) \quad s_{act} = s_{iso}(t)(l_s-l_{CE})/l_{SE0} \tag{11}$$

$$s_f = s_{pass} + s_{act} \qquad \frac{dl_{CE}}{dt} = \left(1-(l_s-l_{CE})/l_{SE0}\right)v_{max}$$

Parameters s_{pass0}, k, l_{s0}, l_{SE0}, v_{max}, and function $s_{iso}(t)$ were derived from physiological experiments on isolated cardiac muscle. From Eq. (11) the length of the contractile element appears an additional state variable, which is solved in the framework of the whole circulation. In Fig. 2 the results of a simulation are shown for occurring pressures and flows in the heart and circulation. Since the hemodynamics of the left ventricle was in focus, a shortcut was made for blood flow from the systemic veins to the mitral valve, thus excluding the pulmonary circulation (Fig. 1).

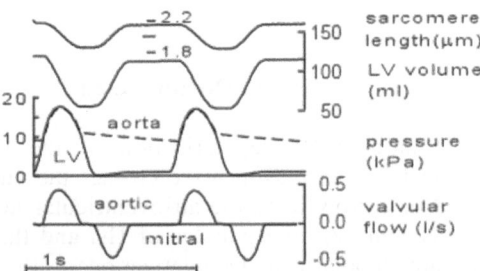

Fig. 2. Simulation of normal hemodynamic variables, using a 1-fiber model of left ventricular mechanics, applying Eq. (10-11).

3.2 Analysis of Cardiac Deformation as Measured with MRI

A method was developed to assess transmural differences in cardiac function. With MRI-tagging motion of the heart can be measured in a number of slices. When imaging two parallel short axis cross-sections near the equator, the most obvious modes of deformation are contraction and torsion. Torsion is defined as a base to apex gradient in rotation angle of the cross-section of the left ventricle around the base to apex axis. Because of the helical structure of the myofibers in the cardiac wall, this torsion contains information about the transmural course of myofiber shortening. The simplest way to model these effects is considering part of the left ventricular wall to be a segment of a cylinder (2, 4). In the model of the whole circulation, the ventricular model can be implemented as follows (Fig. 3). The deformation of the cylinder is a function of left ventricular volume V_{lv}, torsion T, and base to apex length L. Given the length of the contractile elements in the sarcomeres within the wall, stress was calculated (see also Eq. 11). Equilibria of forces are used to solve T and L. Thus, geometry and sarcomere length inside the wall are known. Left ventricular pressure is calculated from the related stresses. Besides, these stresses also determine the time derivatives of contractile element lengths in the wall, which are the state variables associated with the myofibers in the wall. Thus, pressure is a function of volume, and the derivatives of the introduced state variables are known.

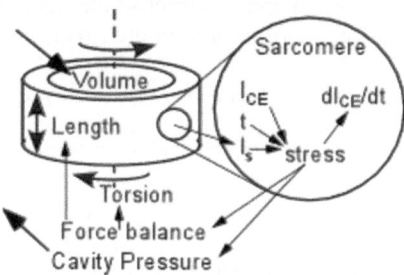

Fig. 3. Pressure as a function of cavity volume. Length and torsion determine sarcomere length l_s. From the resulting stress follows a force balance, to be satisfied by proper choice of torsion and length. Cavity pressure results. Contractile element length l_{CE} is a local state variable, needing its local derivative.

3.3 Sequence of Mechanical Activation During Pacing

Normally, a heartbeat initiated by depolarization of the sinoatrial node (SA). Subsequently, an electrical depolarization wave crosses the atria. With some delay, the wave travels through a narrow duct, the atrioventricular node, thus reaching the ventricular conduction system. Via the bundles of His and the Purkinje conduction system, the ventricles are depolarized. Depolarization of the cardiac cell initiates contraction of the myofibers. So, the sequence of electrical depolarization is reflected in the sequence of mechanical contraction. One of the strategies to obtain non-invasively the sequence of cardiac activation is the measurement of cardiac deformation, followed by a reconstruction. For this reconstruction, a model of cardiac mechanics is used.

To simulate the sequence of electrical (6) and mechanical activation, the heart should be modeled in 3 dimensions. Conventionally the deformation of an object is solved numerically by the finite element method (FEM) (3, 5). With this technique, forces are exerted to the nodes of the mesh. Deformation of the heart is adapted numerically by iteration until the equilibrium of forces is satisfied. So, for a known pressure load, geometry and cavity volume are calculated. Unfortunately, this condition is not compatible with our model setup for the circulation, because pressure should be calculated as a function of volume. A regular solution to this problem is iteration of pressure until FEM-volume V_{FEM} fits the volume V_{lv} in the circulation model (Fig. 4). Such an approach is however very time consuming, because the FEM is incorporated in the iteration. Alternatively, one may use the 1-fiber model (Eq. 10-11) to accurately predict left ventricular pressure. The difference between V_{FEM} and V_{lv} can be used to adjust the parameters of the 1-fiber model to get still better estimates for left ventricular pressure. Correction parameters may be implemented as state variables to be integrated in time.

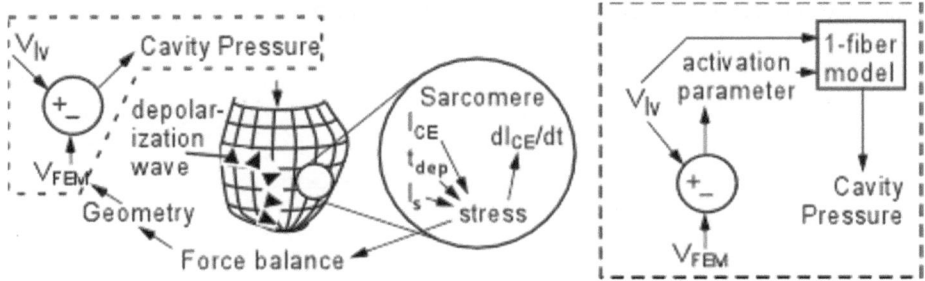

Fig. 4. Implementation of a FEM model of cardiac mechanics in the circulation model. cavity pressure should be described as a function of cavity volume V_{lv}. The FEM model generates volume as a function of pressure. The problem can be solved, either by iteration (left) or using a 1-fiber model, replacing the FEM, while adjusting the 1 fiber model by feedback.

4   Conclusions

A model of the circulation can be used conveniently to harbor modules describing heart mechanics. The structure of the circulation model is a graph network with cavities as nodes and flow ducts as edges. The cavities contain volume as a state variable for the governing set of differential equations. In focussing on various aspects of heart or circulatory dynamics, tailored modules can be inserted, while maintaining overall structure of the model. A toolkit of modules may be extended flexibly.

References

1. Arts T, Bovendeerd PHM, Prinzen FW, and Reneman RS. Relation between left ventricular cavity pressure and volume and systolic fiber stress and strain in the wall. *Biophys J* 59: 93-103, 1991.
2. Arts T, Veenstra PC, and Reneman RS. A model of the mechanics of the left ventricle. *Ann Biomed Eng* 7: 299-318, 1979.
3. Bovendeerd PHM, Arts T, Delhaas T, Huyghe JM, Van Campen DH, and Reneman RS. Regional wall mechanics in the ischemic left ventricle: numerical models and dog experiments. *Am J Physiol* 270: H398-H410, 1996.
4. Chadwick RS. Mechanics of the left ventricle. *Biophys J* 39: 279-288, 1982.

5. Costa KD, Hunter PJ, Wayne JS, Waldman LK, Guccione JM, and McCulloch AD. A three-dimensional finite element method for large elastic deformations of ventricular myocardium: II--Prolate spheroidal coordinates. *J Biomech Eng* 118: 464-72., 1996.
6. Franzone PC, Guerri L, Pennacchio M, and Taccardi B. Spread of excitation in 3-D models of the anisotropic cardiac tissue. II. Effects of fiber architecture and ventricular geometry. *Math Biosci* 147: 131-71., 1998.
7. Noble MIM, Milne ENC, Goerke RJ, Carlsson E, Domenach RJ, Saunders KB, and Hoffman JIE. Left ventricular filling and diastolic pressure-volume relations in the conscious dog. *Circ Res* 24: 269-283, 1969.
8. Sagawa K. The ventricular pressure volume diagram revisited. *Circ Res* 43: 677-687, 1978.
9. Suga H, and Yamakoshi KI. Effect of stroke volume and velocity of ejection on end-systolic pressure of canine left ventricle. *Circ Res* 40: 445-450, 1977.

Geometrical Modeling of the Heart and Its Main Vessels

Jean-Luc Mari, Laurent Astart, and Jean Sequeira

Laboratoire d'Informatique de Marseille, Université de la Méditerranée
Marseille, France
{jlmari, lastart, jsequeira}@esil.univ-mrs.fr

Abstract. This paper introduces a global geometrical modeling approach to represent the heart and its main vessels. It takes into account that this model will be used for heart motion analysis: we have emphasized the role of organ structures because they should be a support for motion representation. But heart and vessels refer to different types of structures: thus, we have defined two different geometrical modeling approaches to handle these two anatomical elements.

Keywords. 3D medical imaging, heart motion modeling, reconstruction

1 Introduction

Geometrical modeling of the heart and its main vessels is required as a support for analyzing their motion. In this paper, we suppose that a segmentation process has been performed and has produced a binary volume, our goal being to associate a geometrical model to it.

An organ can be fully represented by the closed surface that bounds it. This representation is more synthetic than a volumetric description, but we may want to know easily if a given point is located inside or outside the organ: the geometrical model must facilitate the answer to this question.

The geometrical model must also give indications on the organ's topology and morphology, and especially on its structure, such as on its local variation properties.

The modeling approaches we propose to reconstruct the heart and its main vessels satisfy these constraints.

2 Heart Modeling

2.1 Our First Approach

Our first goal was to characterize the global shape of the heart through its structure. For this reason, we have decided to orient our research work towards models based on implicit surfaces, their skeleton giving interesting information on their morphology.

T. Katila et al. (Eds.): FIMH 2001, LNCS 2230, pp. 10-16, 2001.

The reconstruction process is based on the use of the medial axis [1] as a potential source. A specific potential is attached to each point of the medial axis so that the sum of these potentials provides equipotential surfaces [2,3], and especially one surface which has to represent the binary volume's crust as well as possible [4].

The potential function [5] depends on three parameters r, R and k that completely characterize it. Its description is given on Fig. 1.

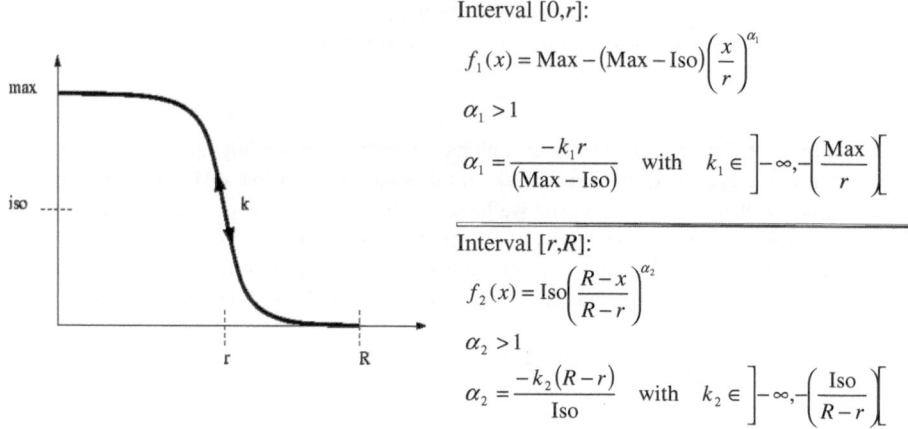

Interval $[0,r]$:

$$f_1(x) = \text{Max} - (\text{Max} - \text{Iso})\left(\frac{x}{r}\right)^{\alpha_1}$$

$$\alpha_1 > 1$$

$$\alpha_1 = \frac{-k_1 r}{(\text{Max} - \text{Iso})} \quad \text{with} \quad k_1 \in \left]-\infty, -\left(\frac{\text{Max}}{r}\right)\right]$$

Interval $[r,R]$:

$$f_2(x) = \text{Iso}\left(\frac{R-x}{R-r}\right)^{\alpha_2}$$

$$\alpha_2 > 1$$

$$\alpha_2 = \frac{-k_2(R-r)}{\text{Iso}} \quad \text{with} \quad k_2 \in \left]-\infty, -\left(\frac{\text{Iso}}{R-r}\right)\right]$$

Fig. 1. The potential function and its formal definition

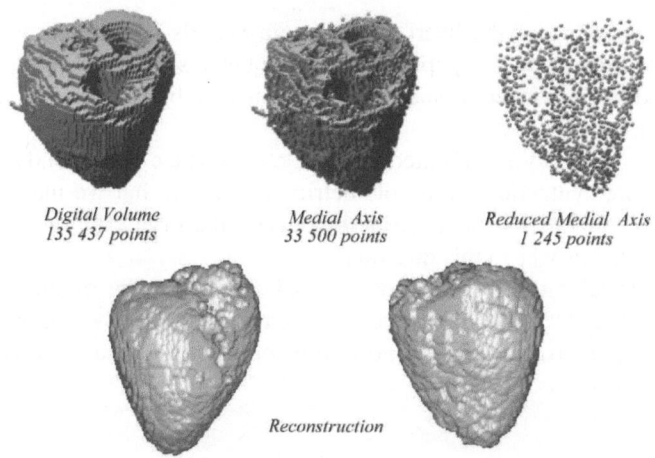

Digital Volume   Medial Axis   Reduced Medial Axis
135 437 points   33 500 points   1 245 points

Reconstruction

Fig. 2. The digital volume of a fetus' heart, the medial axis, its reduction and the reconstruction by implicit surfaces

The reconstruction process consists in determining the set of parameters that minimizes a given energetic criterion. This criterion characterizes the similarity between the equipotential surface and the crust of the binary volume. The entire process is described in [6]. Fig. 2 shows an example of a heart reconstruction based on this approach. The delay for the reconstruction process is about 10 minutes on a 450MHz Pentium III processor (512 Mo RAM). It seems to be satisfactory within a medical examination.

Such a geometrical model provides a surface and volume description (the volume is obtained by the value of the global potential). It also provides an interesting data compression, but two problems rise from this approach:

- the number of potential sources is too high, even after medial axis reduction
- there is no structure underlying the set of potential sources

We found a solution to these two problems through a multilevel approach which is based on the same principles but takes into account strong structural elements.

2.2   A Multilevel Approach

In order to find the binary volume's structure, we have analyzed this data set through different levels of resolution. The first level, which is very rough, provides the global structure of the shape. In fact, the result is made of a few points and it is easy to determine the structure of such a data set (although it is not explicitly used in the reconstruction process). This set of "inner" potential sources gives a basic volume that will be covered and enriched by refining the resolution and completing the external layer. Fig. 3 illustrates this process on a simple example. Each case refers to a sub-resolution of the starting digital volume, strictly included in the latter. The object is seen as a set of layers, in order of structural importance.

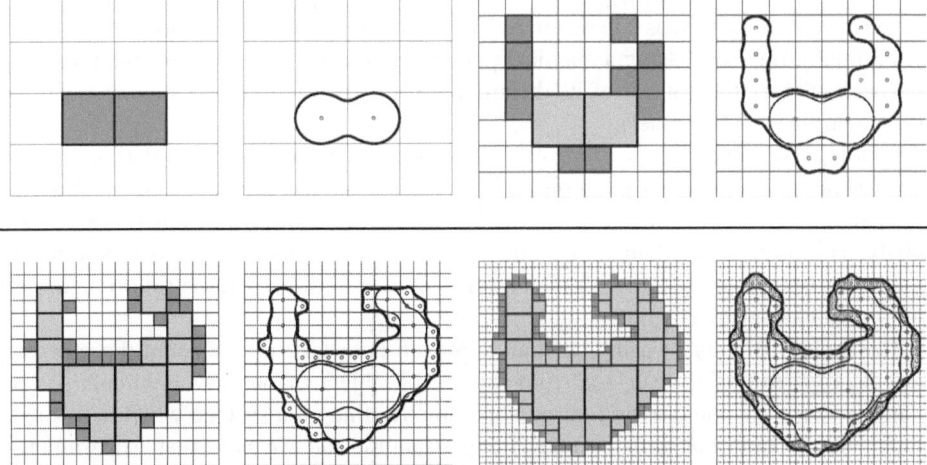

Fig. 3. The layers of an object's model

This multilevel approach is very powerful for many reasons:

- it provides an efficient data compression;
- it gives a representation of both surface and volume;
- it enables the understanding of the heart structure through different layers and skeletons (each one of them is related to a specific layer);

- it provides an interesting support for motion analysis because motion can be split up into complementary components (global motion associated with the inner structure, etc.).

3 Vascular Structure Modeling

The approach described in the previous section cannot be efficiently used for vascular structure modeling because it does not reflect an over structure related to the global orientation of vessels (tree-like structure). Thus, we have developed a complementary model to represent such specific anatomical structures.

3.1 Characterization of a Tree-Like Free-Form Surface

Most of the research work done in this field describes the global surface using a set of patches with conditions on their boundary so as to obtain a given level of continuity globally [7,8,9,10,11].

We have chosen a different approach that consists in using a single parametric patch on which we set topological and morphological conditions.

3.2 Use of a Parametric Model

The shape of a surface is characterized through its topological, morphological and differential properties. Using a classical parametric surface as a basis for the modeling approach enables the control of its differential properties (e.g. using a cubic B-Spline surface produces a C^2 model).

Topological properties are controlled through the definition of invalidation areas in the parametric domain: for example, a bounded parametric domain with invalidation areas made of two connected components (i.e. two "holes") is homeomorph to a sphere with three holes. Thus, a tree-like surface with N ending parts is topologically equivalent to a single patch with (N-1) holes, or to a limited parametric domain with (N-1) invalidation areas.

The main difficulty in using such an approach is to take into account the morphological properties of the surface. And this is the object of our developments. As an example, we show the drawing of an isoparametric line on a surface which is a single patch without hole but with an underlying structure and we note that isoparametric lines do not reflect this structure (Fig. 4a). Even on such a very simple example, we would like these isoparametric lines to be associated with sections (Fig. 4b).

We can provide such a morphological control on the surface through an intermediate interface domain level that reflects the tree-like structure through its parameterization.

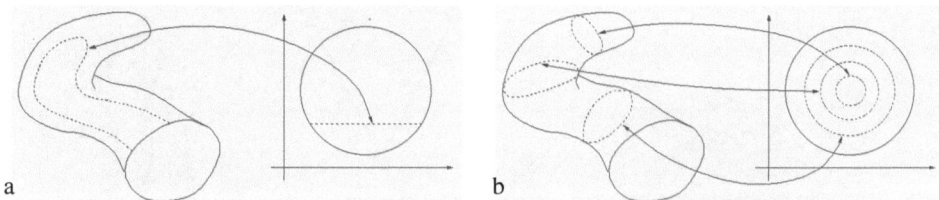

a   b

Fig. 4.   **a.** Image on the surface of an isoparametric line of the definition domain
b. A coherent parameterization of the domain according to the surface

3.3 Need for an Intermediate Interface Level

The final surface can come from any model which uses control points and a classical parameterization. But we do not wish to access directly to these control points to manipulate the surface. Instead, we define an intermediate level of domain with another parameterization. Then, the surface defined by this intermediate level is used to sample the final surface's control points.

Let us consider a junction (the simplest tree-like structure) as an illustration of our approach. The parametrical domain has two invalidation areas that are obtained through the definition of potential sources (we invalidate the areas where the global potential is over a given value, or under another given value). Equipotential lines can then be associated with sections of the junction and provide a new parametric approach (one parameter is defined along these lines and the other in their orthogonal direction), as illustrated on Fig. 5.

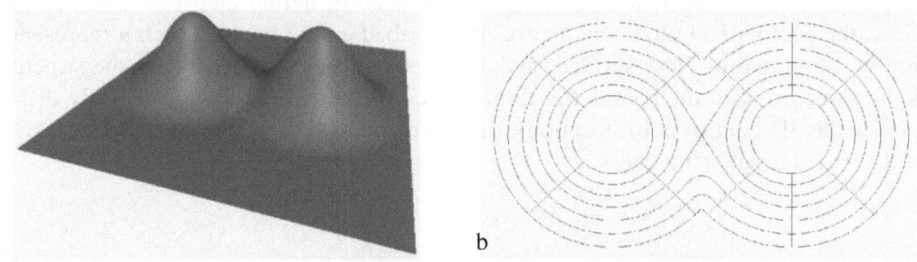

a   b

Fig. 5.   **a.** The parametric domain of a branching shape
b. Isoparametric grid of a branching shape domain

New control points are then obtained through the new parameterization of the intermediate domain. Fig. 6a shows the correspondence between these two levels of control points. We have illustrated our approach through a junction but it is easily generalized to any tree-like structure by associating the basic structure to imbedded potential sources (Fig. 6b shows the structure and Fig. 6c shows the potential value that is used to produce the new parametric domain). Fig. 6d illustrates the use of the model for a vascular structure.

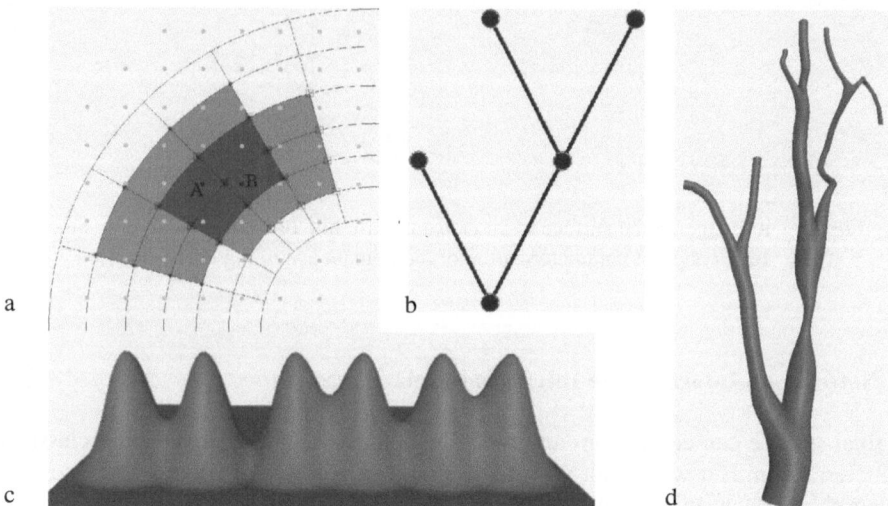

Fig. 6.   **a.** Computation of the control points from the meta control points grid
b. Tree-like free-form surface of a branching shape
c. Parametric domain related to the structure in b
d. Example of a vascular structure

4 Results and Future Work

These two approaches are complementary and well adapted to each case (heart and vessels). Because vessels are not surfaces, we need to define their two walls as surfaces: the geometrical modeling approach described earlier enables such a representation by using two of these surfaces and a correspondence between them (the structure is the same, as with the parametric field and control point definition, the only difference is the 3D control point location), this correspondence facilitating the description of the vessel tissue's thickness.

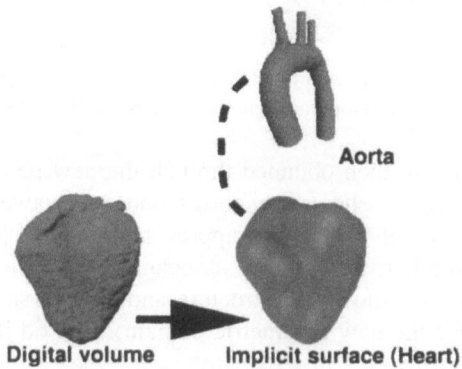

Fig. 7. Heart's data, its reconstruction with implicit surfaces and aorta model

These two geometrical modeling approaches are also interesting for motion description because we can try to analyze and to encode this information at different levels (structural level, surface level). This could be done by making a link with a physical animated model of the heart. Thus, one aim would be to compute functional parameters such as the myocardial mass or the volume variation through time.

One of the remaining problems - and it is a main research axis for us - is the study of the global model's coherence, especially at their junction (aorta, for example) or when they are in contact (coronaries, for example).

Acknowledgments. The authors would like to thank Emilie Lucas for her reading of this paper.

This work was performed within the framework of the joint incentive action "Beating Heart" of the research groups ISIS, ALP and MSPC of the French National Center for Scientific Research (CNRS). It is partly granted by the Lipha Santé Company, a subsidiary of the group MERCK KGaA.

References

1. E. Remy, E. Thiel. Computing 3D medial axis for chamfer distances. In 9th DGCI, Discrete Geometry for Computer Image, volume 1953 of Lectures Notes in Computer Science, pp. 418-430, Uppsala, Sweden, December 2000.
2. S. Muraki. Volumetric shape description of range data using "Blobby Model". Computer Graphics (Proceedings of SIGGRAPH'91), 25(4):227--235, 1991.
3. V.V. Savchenko, A.A. Pasko, O.G. Okunef, T.L.Kunii. Function representation of solids reconstructed from scattered surface points and contours. Eurographics'95, 1995.
4. E. Bittar, N. Tsingos, M.-P. Gascuel. Automatic reconstruction of unstructured 3D data: Combining a medial axis and implicit surfaces. Computer Graphics Forum (Eurographics'95 Proc.), 14:457-468, 1995.
5. C. Guiard. Modèles de surfaces déformables définis et contraints par un ensemble d'informations structurelles. PhD thesis, Université de la Méditerranée - Aix-Marseille II, 2000.
6. J.-L. Mari and J. Sequeira. Using implicit surfaces to characterize shapes within digital volumes. RECPAD 2000 Proceedings, pp. 285-289, Porto, Portugal, May 2000.
7. R. Ebel. Reconstruction interactive d'éléments anatomiques à l'aide de surfaces de forme libre, PhD thesis, E.N.S.T., January 1991.
8. C. Guiard. Etude de la G1 continuité d'embranchements de cylindres généralisés, Master thesis, Faculté des Sciences de Luminy, June 1995.
9. H. Christiansen, T. Sederberg. Conversion of complex contour line definitions into polygonal element mosaic, ACM Computer Graphics, 2(3), 1978.
10. J. Sequeira, R. Ebel, F. Schmitt. Three-dimensional modeling of tree-like structures, Computerized Medical Imaging and Graphics (Pergamon Press), 17(4-5):333-337, November 1993.
11. J. Sequeira, B. Barsky. Geometrical modeling of anatomical structures, in Medical Image Processing: from pixels to structures, Y. Goussard (Eds.), pp. 141-162, Editions de l'Ecole Polytechnique de Montréal, 1997.

Reconstructing 3D Boundary Element Heart Models from 2D Biplane Fluoroscopy

Henri Veisterä[1,2] and Jyrki Lötjönen[3]

[1] Helsinki University of Technology, P.O.Box 2200, FIN-02015 HUT, Finland
[2] BioMag Laboratory, Helsinki University Central Hospital, FIN-00029 HUS, Finland
hveister@cc.hut.fi
[3] VTT Information Technology, P.O.Box 1206, FIN-33101 Tampere, Finland
Jyrki.Lotjonen@vtt.fi

Abstract. Individual 3D boundary element models can be used in solving inverse problems in electro- and magnetocardiographic measurements. In some cases 3D data, such as Magnetic Resonance (MR) or Computed Tomography (CT) images, are not available. Therefore, it would be useful to be able to use 2D images such as X-ray projections for creating 3D models. The aim of this work was to develop a software package for creating a 3D boundary element heart model from two orthogonal X-ray projections. The biplane fluoroscopy images from a patient are digitized and the images are enhanced with different image processing techniques. The patient heart outline is segmented from the X-ray projections. The outline is compared with virtual X-ray projections created from a prior 3D model segmented from MR images. The difference between the outlines is used to deform the prior model. The quality of the digitized X-ray projections was noticeably improved and thus the heart outline segmentation was facilitated. The deformation method implemented is robust and provides good results even when the source parameters contain errors.

1 Introduction

Individual 3D boundary element models can be used in solving inverse problems in electro- and magnetocardiographic measurements. Many other applications exist for individual 3D models in the medical field. In some cases, Magnetic Resonance (MR) or Computed Tomography (CT) images are not available or the cost of obtaining them is too high. Modalities producing 2D data, such as X-ray projections and ultrasound images are more readily available. Therefore, it would be useful to be able to use these images for creating 3D models.

One or two X-ray projections of an object are usually not enough to reconstruct a 3D object. Several X-ray projections of the same object from different angles are needed to create a good 3D approximation of the object. In CT, hundreds of projections are used. If only a few X-ray projections are used, some *a priori* knowledge can be incorporated to improve the reconstruction accuracy. For human anatomy, the prior knowledge, i.e. a representation of typical human anatomy, can be extracted, for example, from MR volumes. This work is based on a method where a 3D model was reconstructed from two 2D silhouettes using a prior 3D model [1].

T. Katila et al. (Eds.): FIMH 2001, LNCS 2230, pp. 17-23, 2001.

The aim of this work was to develop an easy to use software package for creating a 3D heart model from two orthogonal X-ray projections. In addition, 3D model coordinates can be displayed on the original X-ray projections in 2D for persons who are used to locating objects from X-ray projections. Also, 2D coordinates, such as catheter locations, can be visualized with the 3D model.

The developed application is not limited to creating only heart models but it can be applied more generally. Once a prior model of an object and two images of a new slightly different instance of the object are available, this application can be used to reconstruct the 3D geometry of the object.

2 Methods

The geometric prior model used in this work was built from MR images. The data volume used here originates from a cardiac cine MR sequence at diastolic phase. The geometric model is built by first segmenting [2] and then triangulating [3] the cine MR volume. The segmentation is based on free-form deformation of a geometric and topologic prior model. The model is matched to the edges present in the data volume. After segmentation, a set of points is selected from the segmented volume and the points are linked with each other in such a way that triangles are produced. The Voronoi-Delaunay duality is used in the triangulation. The epicardium and both ventricles are included in the model.

The source images are sequences of X-ray images of the heart of a patient, taken at two different orthogonal angles. The images used in this work are taken during catheter operations and contain, in addition to the anatomical features, the electrodes and catheters used during the operation. The images are converted from analog video data into digital format with an image grabbing system.

In order to improve the low quality of the source images, a number of image-processing algorithms were implemented. The source image frames are combined with intelligent averaging to reduce the image noise and interleaving to enhance the resolution. A specifically modified local contrast enhancement algorithm is applied, where the nature (for example, the constant black border) of the source images is taken into account. Local image neighborhood statistics are compared with global statistics and pixel intensities are modified to increase local contrast. The improvement in image quality helps the segmentation and visual inspection of the image. An example of the image enhancement is displayed in (Fig. 1).

Several methods have been proposed for automatic segmentation of X-ray projections, such as active contour models [4] and united snakes [5]. The quality and type of the source images, used in this work, makes them very difficult for automatic segmentation. The problem is further complicated by the fact that the object is often seen only partially in the images. A method, introduced in [1], tries to overcome these problems using prior model information and elastic matching. However, this method has not yet been tried for the type of source images used in this work. The final segmentation of the heart outline is done manually by looking at the pre-processed source image.

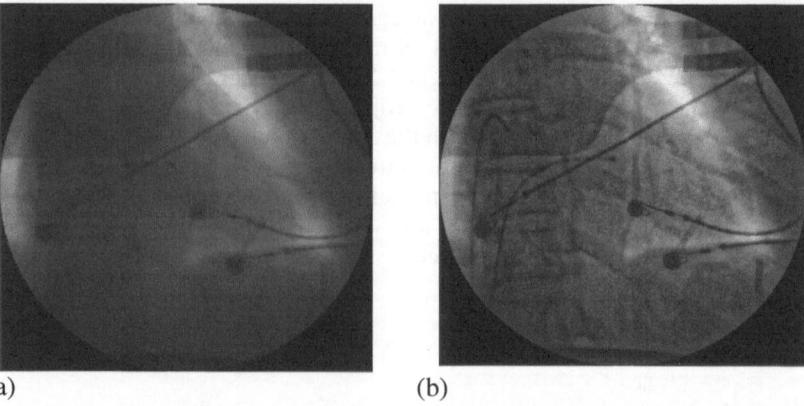

(a)   (b)

Fig. 1. Image enhancement: (a) Original digitized fluoroscopy image; (b) Image processed with frame interleaving, image averaging and local contrast enhancement. The anatomic features in the image and the catheters are now more clearly visible.

The outline is compared with virtual X-ray projections created from a prior 3D model, carefully segmented from MR images of the heart. The 2D vectors generated by matching the actual outlines with the prior model outlines are back-projected onto the 3D model surface. Vectors are interpolated for each model surface point. The original model points are moved according to the displacement vectors. The ventricles of the heart, not visible in the X-ray projections used, are deformed using local scaled averages of the deformations calculated for the epicardium (Fig. 2).

As a result of the previous stages, necessary information exists to map 3D coordinates back to the original 2D projection coordinates. This information can be used to display 3D points on the original 2D projections, for example, on the ventricle surfaces, such as Josephson points. The points can be color-coded to display additional information. Also, 2D coordinates, such as catheter tip locations, on the original projections can be visualized in 3D with the new model (Fig. 3).

3   Results

The quality of the digitized X-ray projections was noticeably improved and thus the heart outline segmentation was facilitated (Fig. 1). At this point the relevant features of the image are considerably more prominent than in the original X-ray image.

The direct validation of the results with actual cases where both 2D silhouette images of the heart and otherwise generated 3D images of the heart could not be done since no such data was available. However, the results can be indirectly observed with just 3D data available. Silhouette images can be generated from the 3D data in various ways, for example, with virtual X-ray projections. These 2D images can then be used to generate 3D models with this application and the deformed models can then be compared with the original models. Such a comparison has been carried out for torso models in [1], where the mean error for the torso models generated was found to be approximately 1.2 voxels for a 128 x 128 x 100 volume. However, the geometric accuracy of the model is not very critical in this work, since the deformed 3D model is inspected only visually.

20   H. Veisterä and J. Lötjönen

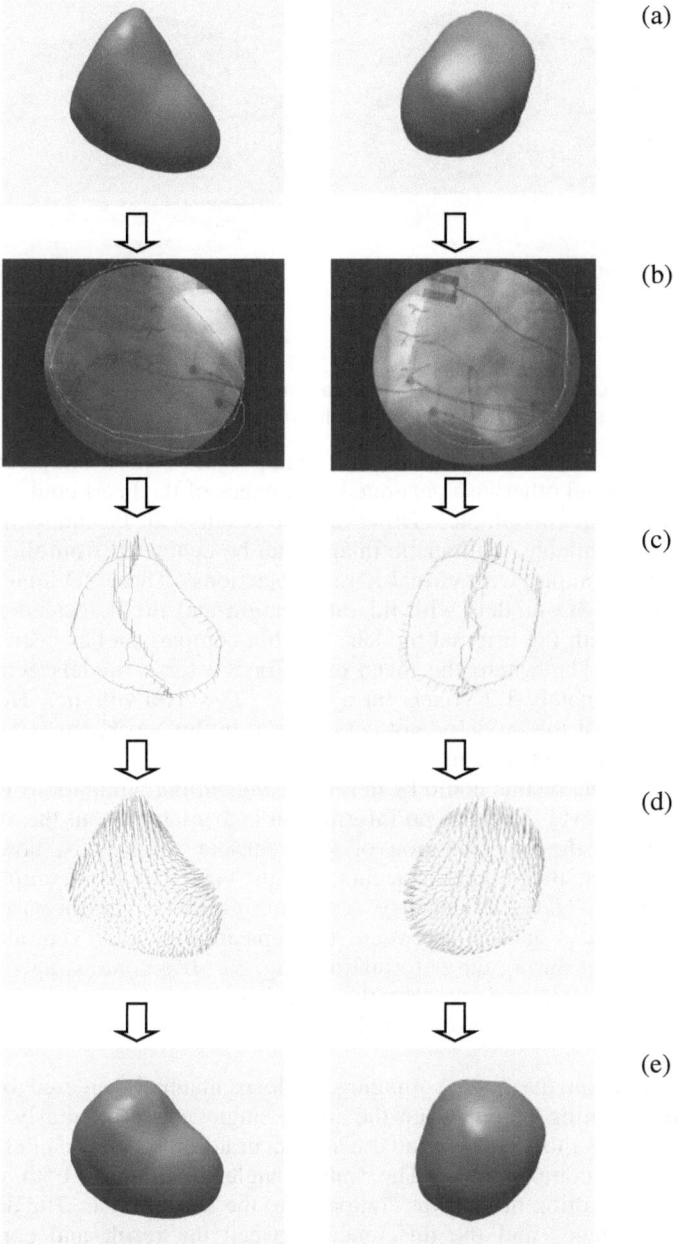

Fig. 2. The deforming process: (a) The original heart model displayed from two orthogonal angles; (b) The patient X-rays where the new heart outline is segmented from. The outlines are compared with virtual X-rays of the original model; (c) The 2D vectors generated from elastic matching between the actual outlines and the model outlines are moved onto the 3D model surface; (d) Vectors are interpolated for each model surface point; (e) The new deformed model.

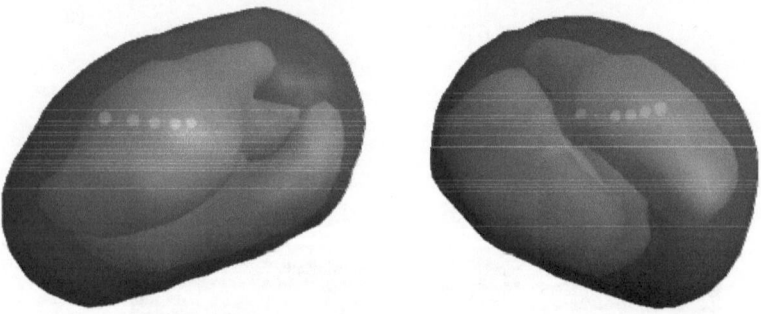

Fig. 3. Two orthogonal views of catheter tip locations digitized from 2D fluoroscopy images visualized in 3D with a heart model including the heart ventricles.

The direct validation of the results with actual cases where both 2D silhouette images of the heart and otherwise generated 3D images of the heart could not be done since no such data was available. However, the results can be indirectly observed with just 3D data available. Silhouette images can be generated from the 3D data in various ways, for example, with virtual X-ray projections. These 2D images can then be used to generate 3D models with this application and the deformed models can then be compared with the original models. Such a comparison has been carried out for torso models in [1], where the mean error for the torso models generated was found to be approximately 1.2 voxels for a 128 x 128 x 100 volume. However, the geometric accuracy of the model is not very critical in this work, since the deformed 3D model is inspected only visually.

The accuracy of the results could be defined using similar simulations to the paper [1], as mentioned above. Because no information is available about the ventricles in X-ray images used, the interpretation of the ventricle surfaces is, however, only qualitative. Therefore, the geometric accuracy of the ventricles is not emphasized and studied in this work. Nevertheless, it is worth noting that since the prior model is used, the geometric relations between the epicardium and ventricles remain approximately correct during the deformation (Fig. 3). If a contrast agent is applied during the catheter operation, so that the ventricle becomes visible in the X-ray projections, a more accurate model of the ventricle can be reconstructed with the software.

The information on the source imaging angle is manually entered by the user. Changes in the resulting output when the source angles are erroneously entered are shown in Table 1. A model was created using accurate orthogonal angles and it was set as the base for comparisons. The source angles for one or both views were modified and the resulting model was compared to the base model. The difference in entered and real angles and the difference between the result and correct object volume is displayed in the table along with the overlap for the result and correct volumes. When the patient heart corresponds well to the used original heart model, the method is very robust to errors in determining the source image angles. Since the goal of the model creation is to reconstruct the correct model shape and not the size, the actual simulation parameters need not closely correspond to the actual X-ray imaging parameters used in the source X-ray projections. The generated model can be easily scaled using, for example, information from ultrasound images.

Table 1. Changes in produced 3D model volume with different source imaging angles

Angle difference	Volume difference	Volume overlap
1°	+0.043 %	99.2 %
2°	+0,061 %	99.2 %
10°	-0,034 %	98.2 %
20°	+0,040 %	97.8 %

The deformation method implemented is robust and provides good results even when the source parameters contain errors. The application is easy to use and new models can be created on-line with a common desktop PC. Currently the software is used to create individual anatomic heart models. However, the software is not limited to creating just heart models.

4 Discussion

Presently, only one object outline can be displayed and edited at one time. If multiple object outlines could be edited at the same time, this would simplify and speed up handling of multiple objects. Also, the relations between the objects could be more easily viewed and edited.

Manual segmentation works well in practice and it can be accomplished in a few minutes. Automatic segmentation such as outlined in [1] could be implemented and tested. However, the visibility of the edges of interest in our images is much poorer than in the thorax-images used in [1]. Moreover, strong edges produced by catheters may distort automatic segmentation. A form of snakes [5] was used to segment the images but this relays heavily on the initial guess for the heart outline to be quite close to the actual outline for acceptable results. Snakes can however be used to segment the heart outline at different phases semi-automatically once the initial segmentation from one frame is accomplished.

Only X-ray images were used as source images but other imaging modalities such as ultra sound imaging where the object silhouette can be seen could be used. Any 2D image where the object silhouette can be observed could be used as a source image. Possible changes in the imaging geometry should be taken into consideration.

An option for increasing the number of source projections could be implemented. In cases, where more projections are available, a more accurate model could be generated using all available data.

References

1.   Lötjönen J., Magnin I. E., Reinhardt L., Nenonen J., Katila T.: Automatic Reconstruction of 3D Geometry Using 2D Projections and a Geometric Prior Model. Lecture Notes in Computer Science 1679: Medical Image Computing and Computer-Assisted Intervention, MICCAI99, C. Taylor, A. Colchester (Eds.), Springer (1999) 192-201

2. Lötjönen J., Reissman P.-J., Magnin I. E., Katila T.: Model Extraction from Magnetic Resonance Volume Data Using the Deformable Pyramid. Medical Image Analysis (1999) 3 387-406
3. Lötjönen J., Reissman P.-J., Magnin I. E., Nenonen J., Katila T.: A Triangulation Method of an Arbitrary Point Set for Biomagnetic Problems. IEEE Trans. Magn (1998) 34 2228-2233
4. Gerard O., Makram-Ebeid S.: Automatic Contour Detection by Encoding Knowledge into Active Contour Models. Proceedings Fourth IEEE Workshop on Applications of Computer Vision (WACV'98) (1998) 115-120
5. Liang J., McInerney T., Terzopoulos D.: Interactive Medical Image Segmentation with United Snakes. Lecture Notes in Computer Science 1679: Medical Image Computing and Computer-Assisted Intervention, MICCAI99, C. Taylor, A. Colchester (Eds.), Springer (1999) 116-127

Introducing Spectral Estimation for Boundary Detection in Echographic Radiofrequency Images

Igor Dydenko, Denis Friboulet, and Isabelle E. Magnin

CREATIS, INSA - Blaise Pascal, F - 69621 Villeurbanne Cedex
dydenko@creatis.insa-lyon.fr

Abstract. In echocardiography, the radio-frequency (RF) image is a rich source of information about the investigated tissues. Nevertheless, very few works are dedicated to boundary detection based on the RF image, as opposed to envelope image. In this paper, we investigate the feasibility and limitations of boundary detection in echocardiographic images based on the spectral contents of the RF signal. Using the system approach, we study on models and simulations how the spectral contents can be used for boundary detection. We then introduce an original method of spectral estimation for boundary detection, and several images are analyzed with its mean. It is shown that, under the condition of high acquisition frequency, it is possible to use the spectral contents for boundary detection, and that improvement can be expected with respect to traditional methods. The conclusions may enable development of a robust boundary detection method, based both on the envelope and the spectral contents of the RF signal.

1 Introduction

The interest of echography is well known. As compared to other medical imaging methods it is a relatively low-cost, fast and non-invasive method. Applied to the cardiac field, it enables real time imaging of the heart. In the perspective of accurate assessment of the cardiac function, automatic boundary detection in echographic images appears as a key issue. This problem has been widely treated in literature, however, due to speckle noise and image artifacts, it still remains a challenging and open problem.

The unprocessed radio-frequency (RF) signal from the ultrasound scanner is potentially rich in information about the investigated organ and the boundaries between tissues. Recent works in echography successfully use spectrum analysis of RF signals to characterize the explored tissues [1] [2]. However, none of those works apply spectrum analysis to boundary detection, which continues to be performed almost exclusively on envelope (B-scan) images (see for example [3]). Such images are obtained by demodulating the RF signal, and its spectral contents is lost in this process.

In the current paper, we address the feasibility of boundary detection based on the spectral contents of the RF signal. With a Discontinuity Adaptive method

T. Katila et al. (Eds.): FIMH 2001, LNCS 2230, pp. 24–31, 2001.

of spectral estimation introduced by us in [6], we investigate the advantages and limitations of such an approach, as compared to traditional methods based exclusively on the envelope of the signal. This work is carried out in view of its application to the field of cardiac imaging.

2   Boundary Detection Method

Due to the stochastic nature of the RF signal, exploring its spectral contents requires a spectral estimation method, and consequently, choosing appropriate spectral parameters: discrepancy between such parameters issued from different tissues will enable correct boundary detection. It has been proposed in [4] to model portions of the RF signal as an autoregressive (AR) process of order p, characterized by the variance σ^2 of the driving noise and the reflection coefficients γ_k. Such a description is equivalent to the Power Spectrum Density (PSD) [5]. We have introduced in [6] an original method, combining spectral AR (parametric) estimation with Discontinuity Adaptive (DA) smoothing. Other works in this area [4] [12] do not take into account discontinuities while smoothing, and therefore are less suitable for the task of recovering boundaries. Our method can be directly applied to boundary detection, based both on the envelope and on the spectral contents of the echographic RF image. We briefly recall the method here, and apply it in section 5 to detect boundaries on several echographic images.

The RF signal along each acquisition line is partitioned into short windows. At each consecutive AR order k we adopt the following two-step algorithm: (I) the reflection coefficients of order k (γ_k) are estimated for all the windows of the image using the Burg iterative scheme, (II) based on the field Γ_k of coefficients γ_k, the smoothed field $\tilde{\Gamma}_k$ is obtained by means of a DA method. This second step is essential in the context of boundary detection. The solution $\tilde{\Gamma}_k$ is obtained by minimizing a cost function of the form:

$$C(\hat{\Gamma}_k \mid \Gamma_k) = \sum_{\forall s} \alpha_s \parallel \hat{\gamma}_k^s - \gamma_k^s \parallel^2 + \eta \sum_{s,t \in V} \Phi(\hat{\gamma}_k^s - \hat{\gamma}_k^t) \tag{1}$$

The first term stands for data fidelity, where we consider the field Γ_k as the observation data. The second term takes into account the smoothness constraint, formalized through Markovian Random Fields applied on a neighborhood V. A non quadratic Φ-function results in smoothing relatively even areas of the image, while preserving discontinuities [7] [8]. The parameter η is a weighting term which tunes the conditions of smoothing. We use an equivalent description of the Φ-function, based on the so-called dual fields [8]. We thus obtain a dual field associated with the smoothed field of coefficients, and it is this very dual field that we regard as a map of discontinuities.

3   Theoretical Modeling

We model the RF signal formation process by the system approach, largely used in literature [10] [11] [9]. The PSD of the RF image $|I(f,p)|^2$ at the observed point p is obtained by the multiplication of two terms: the pulse response at the focal point $|H(f)|^2$ and the tissue response $|T(f,p)|^2$:

$$|I(f,p)|^2 = |H(f)|^2 \cdot |T(f,p)|^2 \qquad (2)$$

Backscattering of the tissue is proportional to the 2nd derivative of its acoustic impedance fluctuations in the direction of the wave propagation. In the adopted inhomogeneous continuum approach, the tissue is modeled as an ensemble of gaussian scatterers, randomly distributed in the tissue. The pulse, $H(x,y)$, is described as a cosine wave of central frequency f_0 modulated by a gaussian.

For the purpose of our simulations we define three tissues, determined by the shapes of the scatterers: *(A)* symmetric gaussian shape, of equivalent diameter $d = 150\mu m$, *(B)* gaussian shape oriented at an angle $\phi = 10^0$ of equivalent length $d_l = 100\mu m$ and diameter $d_t = 10\mu m$ and *(C)* very small gaussian scatterers. The corresponding tissue responses are given below, where k is the wave number and the term k^4 stands for the second derivative

$$|T_A(k)|^2 = k^4 \cdot e^{-2k^2 d^2/4} \qquad (3)$$

$$|T_B(k)|^2 = k^4 \cdot e^{-2k^2(d_l^2 \cos^2 \phi + d_t^2 \sin^2 \phi)/4} \qquad (4)$$

Using the same framework, 2D acquisitions can be simulated [11]: 2D tissues corresponding to *A-C* are depicted in Fig. 1. These simulations mimic 3 tissues encountered in cardiac imaging: the external tissue, the cardiac muscle with its oriented fibers and blood with small blood cells. The task of boundary detection in cardiac imaging requires discriminating between such tissues. We simulate two acquisition pulses whose central frequencies f_0 of 2 and 5 MHz approximately correspond to the lower and upper bounds in human echocardiography:

$$|P(f)|^2 = e^{-(f-f_0)^2/\sigma_f^2} \qquad (5)$$

The bandwidth of the pulse, introduced through the parameter σ_f^2, increases with frequency.

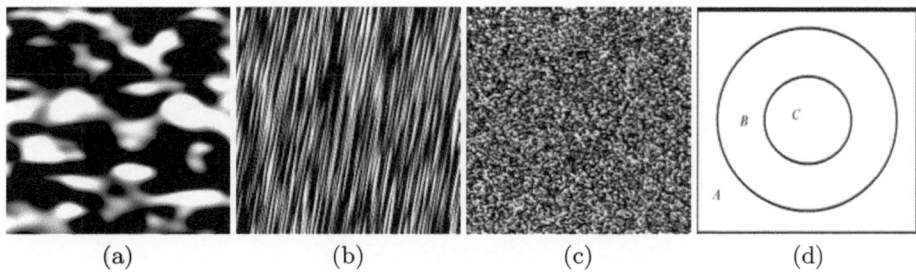

    (a)   (b)   (c)   (d)

Fig. 1. (a) - (c) modeled tissues, corresponding to *A-C* (see text), (d) a scheme specifying the shape of the simulated body and the positions of the tissues

4   Modeling Results

Based on considerations from section 2, theoretical expressions of PSD of the
resulting RF signals are derived. Fig. 2(a), (b) present the PSD of the signals,
each one issued from insonification of one tissue (tissues A, B, C) with the pulse
of 2 MHz and of 5 MHz. The three spectra are almost identical at acquisition
frequency 2 MHz, and much more dissimilar at 5 MHz. Hence, it seems that
segmentation will be much easier in the latter case.

We subsequently simulate echographic imaging of the synthetic body (Fig. 1)
with the two aforementioned pulses, obtaining thus two RF images. In regions
corresponding to each of the tissues we estimate one spectral parameter: the
reflection coefficient of order 1 (γ_1). It is a complex coefficient, whose phase is
dependant on the central frequency of the PSD. The higher the central frequency
of the PSD, the higher the phase of γ_1. Let us also remind that the phase
rises in the anti-clockwise direction in complex coordinates. Due to the non-
stationarity of the signal, estimation is performed on short windows, yielding
several estimates of γ_1. The results are represented in Fig. 2(c), (d) in complex
coordinates. The dispersion of the values inside one population results from the
stochastic nature of the tissue simulation [11], as well as from the process of
numerical estimation itself.

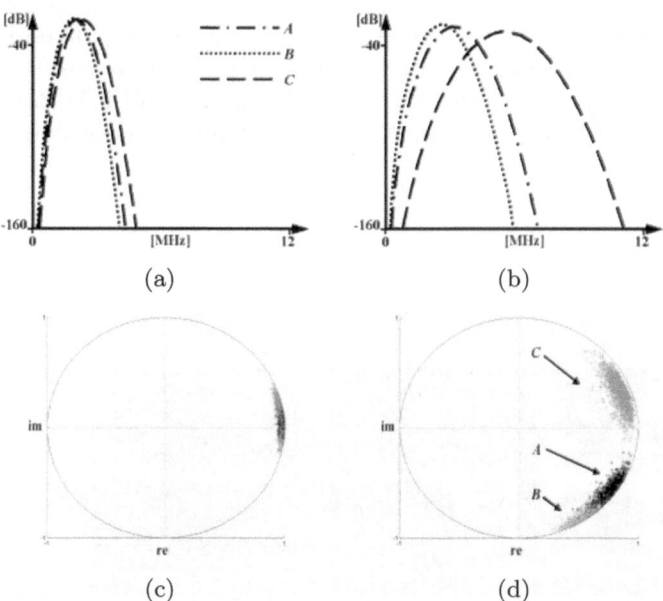

Fig. 2. (a), (b): theoretical spectra (in dB) of RF signals acquired at f_0, respectively, 2
and 5 MHz. (c), (d) 3 populations of coefficient γ_1 represented in complex coordinates,
with complex circle of radius 1, acquired at f_0 2 and 5 MHz

It is clear that the three populations of reflection coefficients are far better distinguishable with an acquisition at higher frequency. This confirms previous observations. Detection of boundaries based on the spectral parameter γ_1 appears feasible for the higher acquisition frequency, while it seems an extremely difficult task for the 2-MHz acquisition.

5   Boundary Detection Results

In order to confirm the observations of section 4, we process echographic images acquired in different conditions: a simulation, a human and a canine heart. For each case, we present several figures: the envelope image; boundaries detected with our DA method based on the envelope image, which corresponds to processing a conventional B-scan image; boundaries detected with our DA method based on the spectral parameter γ_1 and based on the spectral parameter γ_2. Running our DA-method requires adjusting two hyperparameters: the weighting parameter η (see eq. 1) and a threshold parameter δ for the function Φ. For each image separately, we set these hyperparameters so as to obtain optimal results in the sense of a trade-off between noise and actual discontinuities.

The simulation image (see Fig. 3) is issued from insonification of the synthetic body shown in Fig. 1 (simulated transducer on top of the image). Attenuation is taken into account, and the pulse frequency is 7 MHz, which approaches, according to previous remarks, ideal conditions of imaging. Acoustic parameters of the tissues have been intentionally chosen so that the contrast of the envelope image is very poor. As a consequence, the result based on the envelope is unsatisfactory: merely half of the initial contour is recovered. A different choice of the hyperparameters does not reveal new contours, but only artifacts, mainly due to attenuation. It is the introduction of the spectral contents through the complex reflection coefficient γ_1 that enables correct detection of actual boundaries, with relatively few artifacts. Therefore, in this particular situation, the use of the spectral contents appears to be necessary for correct boundary detection.

The image of the human heart, acquired at 2 MHz over 106 acquisition lines, shows a long axis view of the left ventricle (see Fig. 4). Low acquisition fre-

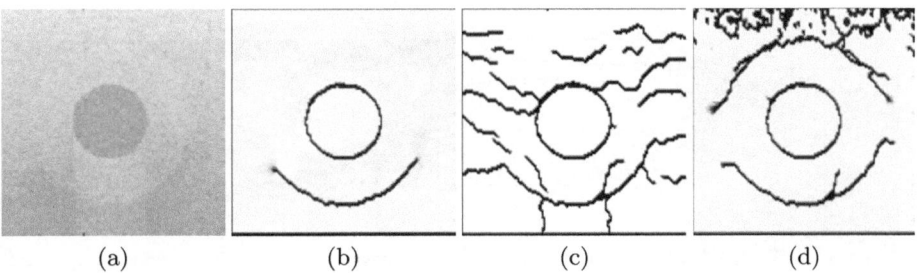

(a)   (b)   (c)   (d)

Fig. 3. Simulation image: (a) envelope, (b) boundaries detected based on envelope, (c) boundaries detected based on envelope with sub-optimal choice of hyperparameters, (d) boundaries detected based on γ_1

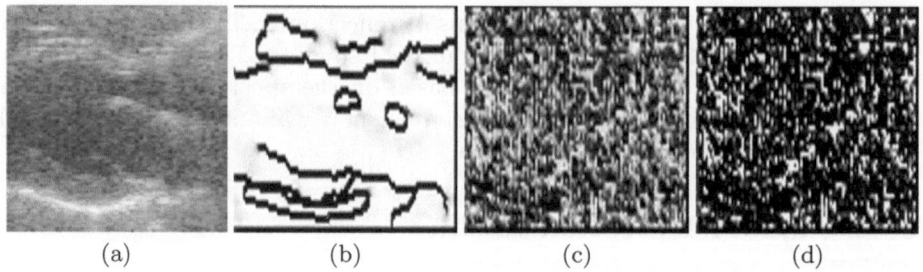

Fig. 4. Human heart: (a) envelope, (b) boundaries detected based on envelope, (c) and (d) boundaries detected based on γ_1 with two different choices of hyperparameters

quency yields a poor visual quality of this image. The envelope enables to detect the internal walls of the cardiac cavities, as well as several cardiac structures. However, detection based on γ_1 gives completely random contours. Conclusions from section 4 are confirmed: at low acquisition frequencies, the spectral contents is irrelevant and there is little hope that it can be used to improve boundary detection.

The image of the canine heart represents a long axis view of the left ventricle acquired at the frequency of 5 MHz over 120 lines (see Fig. 5). Higher acquisition frequency and large acquisition area result in a better image quality. It is worth noting that the structure below the left ventricle is a ghost (mirror) image, and therefore has no medical meaning. When using the envelope, an important part of the heart cavity is properly detected, along with different cardiac structures. Reflection coefficient γ_1 yields some new boundaries, such as closing the left ventricle at the apex. Reflection coefficient γ_2 yields similar results. In this situation, the use of the spectral contents could contribute to accurate detection of contours. Nonetheless, parasite discontinuities appear, especially inside of the cardiac muscle where the spectrum shows very high variability.

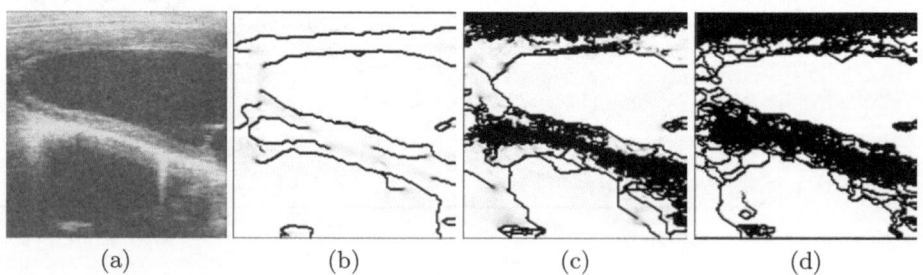

Fig. 5. Canine heart: (a) envelope, (b) boundaries detected based on envelope, (c) boundaries detected based on γ_1, (d) boundaries detected based on γ_2

6   Conclusion and Perspectives

We have proposed to introduce the spectral contents of the RF signal to detect boundaries in echocardiographic images, and we have also described a novel method to perform this task. Results obtained on models, simulations and actual RF images converge towards the same conclusions. For low acquisition frequencies, the spectral parameters estimated from different tissues are not dissimilar enough to become meaningful for boundary detection. Indeed, the estimated parameters are subject to natural variability, due to fluctuations of the acoustic properties inside one tissue, acquisition noise and estimation variability. In the case of higher acquisition frequencies, spectral parameters can successfully be used for detection of discontinuities, and we have shown a simulation case in which the introduction of the spectral contents significantly improves the quality of detected boundaries. We have also proven that complex reflection coefficients, in particular the coefficient of order 1, are suitable spectral parameters for the task of boundary detection. These conclusions open promising ways to improve boundary detection on echographic images. It appears feasible to use the spectral contents to find new boundaries, which are not detected based on the envelope image. It may also be possible to merge boundaries detected based on the envelope and several spectral parameters, providing a measure of confidence affected to the detected boundaries.

The limitation on high frequencies is related to attenuation, which increases with frequency. Therefore, high acquisition frequencies cannot be used for imaging of the human heart, where distances involved are relatively long. Spectrum-based segmentation could be adapted for children (pulse frequencies up to 8 MHz), and also transesophagus (transthoracic) echocardiography, where distances are shorter. Besides, applications other than cardiac can be considered, such as intravascular imaging (pulse frequencies up to 40 MHz).

Acknowledgements. The authors would like to thank Bart Bijnens and Jan D'hooge from the Cardiac Ultrasound Research Group of the Katholieke Universiteit Leuven, Belgium, for acquisition of canine RF images, as well as Fadi Jamal, cardiologist from the Neuro-Cardiologic Hospital of Lyon, France, for acquisition of human RF images.

References

1. F. L. Lizzi, E. J. Feleppa, M. Astor and A. Kalisz. statistics of US spectral parameters for prostate and liver examinations. *IEEE Trans. Ultras. Ferr. Freq. Contr.*, **44**(4): 935-942, 1997.
2. P. Chaturvedi and M. F. Insana. Errors in biased estimators for parametric ultrasonic imaging. *IEEE Trans. Med. Imag.*, **17**(1): 53-61, 1998.
3. M. Mulet-Parada and J. A. Noble. 2D+T acoustic boundary detection in echocardiography. *Med. Im. Anal.*, **4**: 21-30, 2000.

4. J.-F. Giovannelli, G. Demoment and A. Herment. A Bayesian Method for Long AR Spectral Estimation: A Comparative Study. *IEEE Trans. Ultras. Ferr. Freq. Contr.*, **43**(2): 220-232, 1996.

5. S. M. Kay. *Modern Spectral Estimation: theory and application.*, Alan V. Oppenheime, Signal processing series, Englewood Cliffs: Prentice Hall, 1988.

6. J.M. Gorce, D. Friboulet, J. D'hooge, B. Bijnens, and I.E. Magnin. Regularized autoregressive models for a spectral estimation scheme dedicated to medical ultrasonic RF images. *IEEE Intern. Ultras. Symp.*, Toronto (Canada), 1461-1464, 1997.

7. P. Charbonnier, L. Blanc-Feraud, G. Aubert, M. Barlaud. Deterministic edge-preserving regularization in computed imaging. *IEEE Trans. Im. Proc.*, **6**(2): 298-311, 1997.

8. D. Geman, and G. Reynolds. Constrained restoration and the recovery of discontinuities, *IEEE Trans. Pattern Anal. Mach. Intell.*, **14**(3): 367-383, 1992.

9. M. F. Insana and D. G. Brown. Acoustic scattering theory applied to soft biological tissues. In: *Ultrasonic scattering in biological tissues*: 75-124, CRC Press, 1993.

10. R. F. Wagner, M. F. Insana and D. G. Brown. Statistical properties of rf and envelope-detected signals with applications to medical ultrasound. *J. Opt. Soc. Am.*, **4**(5): 910-922, 1987.

11. J. Meunier and M. Bertrand. Echographic image mean gray level changes with tissue dynamics: a system-based model study. *IEEE Trans. Biomed. Eng.*, **42**(4): 403-410, 1995.

12. G. Kitagawa, and W. Guersh. A smoothness priors long ar model method for spectral estimation, *IEEE Trans. Autom. Control*, **30**(1): 57-65, 1985.

Geometrical Modelling of the Fibre Organization in the Human Left Ventricle

Ayman Mourad[1,2], Luc Biard[2], Denis Caillerie[1], Pierre-Simon Jouk[3,4], Annie Raoult[2], Nicolas Szafran[2], and Yves Usson[3]

[1] Laboratoire Sols, Solides, Structures, BP 53, 38041 Grenoble Cedex 9, France
[2] Laboratoire de Modélisation et Calcul/IMAG, BP 53, 38041 Grenoble Cedex 9, France
[3] Laboratoire TIMC, Domaine de de la Merci, 38076 La Tronche Cedex, France
[4] Unité fonctionnelle Biologie du développement et Génétique clinique, CHU, BP 217, 38043 Grenoble Cedex 9, France

Abstract. The aim of the present study is to check, by means of elementary mathematical tools, a conjecture according to which myocardial fibres are geodesic curves running on some surfaces. This conjecture was first stated and experimentally checked by Streeter (1979) for the equatorial part of the left ventricle free wall. Quantitative polarized light microscopy provides measurements on fibre orientation that could lead to evidence that the conjecture remains true for the whole of the left ventricle. Study of the right ventricle is under progress.

1 Introduction

It is commonly believed [3] that the myocardium design and structure allow maximal mechanical efficiency in the systole and diastole processes. The long-term purpose of our multi-disciplinary approach is to try and propose a model for the mechanical behaviour of the myocardium. In the long run, performance of the complete electro-mechanical system could be analyzed. For related works, see [1], [7]. It is well known that usual mechanical models for skeletal muscles are of no help for the myocardium. Obviously, the myocardium is not, as ordinary muscles, linked at both ends to a bone. Fibre micro-structure and fibre geometrical organization are quite different as well. We believe that the specific fibre organization in the myocardium should be taken into account in a complete model. Numerous anatomical studies, see *e.g.* [8], [9], have been devoted along the years to a description of the fibres arrangement and we refer to [5] for an extensive bibliography. What will be sufficient to recall here is that the dissection or peeling techniques are not precise enough, since apparently preferred fibre directions can be inferred by the experimental process. Data have been improved by means of several techniques in microscopy, such as photonic or electronic microscopy. In the present work, we use the data provided by the polarized light microscopy devices developed by some of the authors [4], [5].

More precisely, we intend to check the geometrical description proposed by Streeter [9] who introduced a topological representation of the left ventricle

T. Katila et al. (Eds.): FIMH 2001, LNCS 2230, pp. 32–38, 2001.

as a "nested set of toroidal bodies of revolution" on which myocardial fibres run as geodesics. This information would increase our understanding of the biomechanical properties and propagation of electrical stimuli in the heart.

The experimental technique, which is valid for both ventricles and for the septum, measures for a set of points located on several myocardial sections two angles from which the fibre orientation can be deduced. In other terms, the output of the experimental work is a discrete three-dimensional vector field. Assuming that the left ventricle has a structure of revolution, we use the invariance of Clairaut's constant along geodesics as a first hint that the conjecture might be true.

Work under progress is devoted to a similar description of the right ventricle. Note however that the simple structure of revolution of the left ventricle is no longer true for the right ventricle.

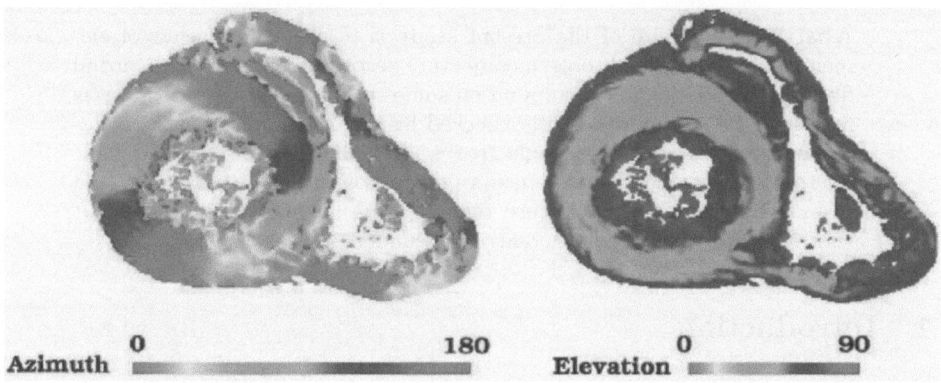

Fig. 1. Maps of the azimuth and elevation angles obtained by means of polarized light microscopy in a coronal section.

2 Data

The data are obtained on fetal hearts. We refer to [4] and [5] for a complete description of the protocol. Let us just recall that the ventricles are embedded in a transparent resin in which they can be clearly seen after polymerization. Sections that can be transversal, sagittal or coronal can then be cut. A section thickness is $500\mu m$, and, because of the thickness of the saw, adjacent sections are separated by a $250\mu m$ gap. The measurement technique relies on the birefringence properties of myocardial cells: in short, the velocity of the light is slower when travelling along the long axis than along the short axis of the fibre. Results are given pointwise: each section is dicretized in $130\mu m \times 130\mu m$ squares, and a mean angular information is collected for each of these elementary squares. For each voxel, the acquisition and representation processes result in two angles:

the angle of elevation γ_{ele} which is the angle between the fibre and the plane of the section, and the azimuth angle γ_{azi} which is the angle between the projection of the fibre on the section plane and a fixed direction in this plane, namely the east-west axis. A local knowledge at point (x, y, z) of these two angles which should range from 0 to π for γ_{azi} and $-\pi/2$ to $\pi/2$ for γ_{ele} determines completely the direction $\boldsymbol{\tau}$ of the fibre

$$\boldsymbol{\tau} = \begin{vmatrix} \tau_x = \cos\gamma_{ele}\cos\gamma_{azi} \\ \tau_y = \cos\gamma_{ele}\sin\gamma_{azi} \\ \tau_z = \sin\gamma_{ele} \end{vmatrix}$$

A drawback of the experimental device in its present state is that it provides the same value for γ_{ele} and $-\gamma_{ele}$. As a consequence and because of the averaging technique, values closed to 0° cannot be reached. Moreover, angles between 75° and 90° cannot be resolved. The accuracy of the method has been checked on myocardial samples which fibres are parallel: the resolution of the measurement method for both angles is 1°.

From a mathematical point of view, we are given a discrete sample of a distributed vector field.

3   Geodesics

According to Streeter [9], in the equatorial part of the left ventricle free wall, fibres are organized into surfaces on which they run as geodesics. In order to check and extend this conjecture to the whole left ventricle, let us first recall some elementary properties of geodesics.

Definition: A regular curve of a given surface of $\mathbf{R}^3$ is a geodesic if and only if its principal normal at any point is normal to the surface.

This definition has well known consequences in terms of lengths [2].

Proposition: Any geodesic locally minimizes the arc length between two points. Conversely, when a regular curve is the shortest path between any two of its points, it is a geodesic.

Note that, in general, an arbitrary geodesic does not minimize globally the arc length between two of its points. For instance, an helix on a vertical cylinder links points on a same vertical line that can be more economically connected through a vertical straight line. Can we expect to find geodesics on any surface? Two answers are well known. First, local existence of a geodesic starting from a given point and tangent to a given vector belonging to the tangent plane at this point is an easy consequence of the fact that a geodesic on a parametrized surface is given by a system of two ordinary differential equations. Second, a global existence result is available in the case of closed surfaces: there exists a minimum geodesic joining two given points of a closed surface (particular case of the Hopf-Rinow theorem, [6]).

In the present study, we assume that the left ventricle has a structure of revolution. Namely, we see the outer surface as generated by rotating a meridian curve, described by Streeter as crescent-shaped, around a vertical axis, see Figure 2. The distance between this generating curve and the axis of revolution is close to 0, but not 0, at the apex which allows fibres to invaginate. Internal layers, if they exist, are also seen as rotation invariant. Computer Aided Design (CAD) approximate models using B-spline smooth surfaces have been constructed. They are out of the scope of the present paper and are used in a parallel work as test models for fibre reconstruction algorithms. This simplifying assumption allows us to use a specific property of geodesics of surfaces of revolution [2].

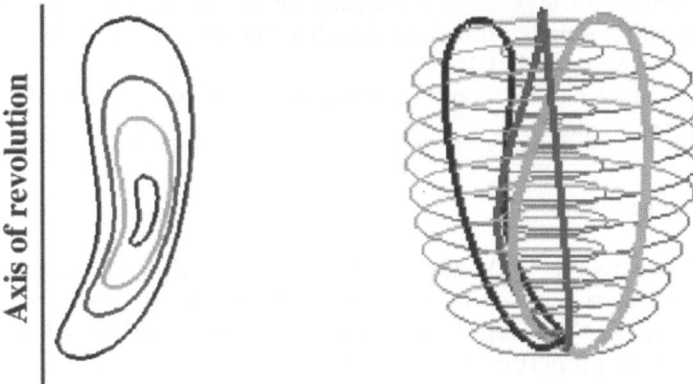

Fig. 2. An ideal setting. Left: nested meridian curves. Right: periodic geodesics deduced one from the other by rotations.

Clairaut's constant: For any point on a curve on a surface of revolution, let r be the distance from this point to the axis of revolution and let θ be the angle between the tangent to this curve and the parallel of the surface at this point. If the curve is a geodesic, then the quantity $r \cos \theta$ remains invariant along the curve. It is called the Clairaut constant.

Note that the above property is not sufficient for a curve to be a geodesic. Along all parallels, *e.g.*, the quantity $r \cos \theta$ remains constant since it is equal to r, but only some of the parallels are geodesics.

4   Experimental Validation

As seems to be true from anatomical observations, assume that the left ventricle fibres are organized in nested toroidal layers with the same axis of revolution and that they are periodic geodesics of these layers, *i.e.*, the fibres follow closed curves with continuous tangents. Furthermore, assume that the fibres on a given layer can be deduced one from the other by rotations around the axis of revolution. Figure 2 describes an ideal setting where the geodesics have been computed on the abstract CAD model (the algorithm numerically solves the system of ordinary differential equations characterizing a geodesic). Then the

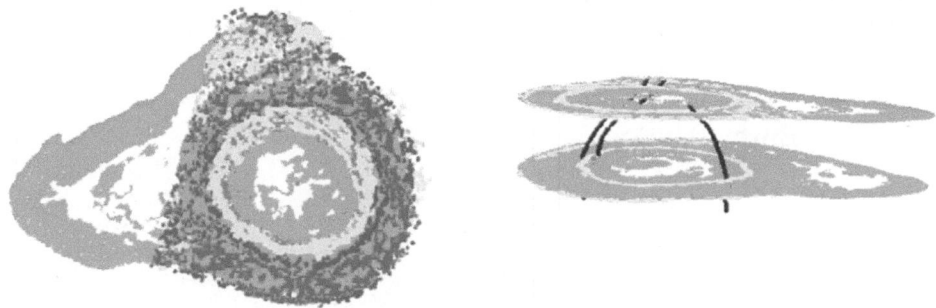

Fig. 3. Left: isovalues of $r\cos\theta$ on a given coronal section. Right: Fibre trajectories crossing traces of a given C on several coronal sections.

Clairaut constant is the same for all fibres in the layer, but may vary from one layer to another. As a consequence, if the conjecture is true, then the isovalues of $r\cos\theta$, where θ denotes here the angle between the vector $\boldsymbol{\tau}$ at point (x, y, z) and the parallel at this same point, will be nested toroidal surfaces. The traces of these surfaces on each coronal section (a section which is orthogonal to the left ventricle axis) should be concentric circles. This comes from the fact that the fibres are supposed to be organized in layers and globally rotationally invariant on each layer. Moreover, a same constant value of $r\cos\theta$ should appear on two separate concentric circles translating the fact that the fibre invaginates and, then, makes at least one complete turn before closing back. As for the trace of each surface of isovalues on a meridian plane, it should consist of two symmetrical closed crescent-shaped curves.

With this in mind, we have computed $r\cos\theta$ for our experimental data. In order to use what is actually provided to us, namely the vector field $\boldsymbol{\tau}$, we have used the obvious identity

$$r\cos\theta = |-y\tau_x + x\tau_y|.$$

We have traced the lines of isovalues on several coronal section planes. We readily observe that on each section they are, as anticipated, concentric circles, and that a same constant value of $r\cos\theta$ appears on two separate concentric circles. In the same time, we have developed an algorithm which follows the fibres from section to section in the whole of the myocardium. By means of an interpolation procedure, the algorithm first transforms the given discrete data into a distributed vector field. Then, for a given h, the iterative procedure constructs a point from the previous one by moving with length h along its vector direction. In the left ventricle, the obtained trajectories cross the circles that correspond to a same Clairaut constant. In parallel, we have traced several isovalues of $r \cos \theta$ on two longitudinal section planes, one orthogonal and the other parallel to the interventricular septum (namely, transversal and sagittal sections), from the apex to the base. The result shows, as expected, a nested set of meridian curves which is similar to the abstract model described in Figure 2.

Clearly, an arbitrary vector field τ would not satisfay the above properties.

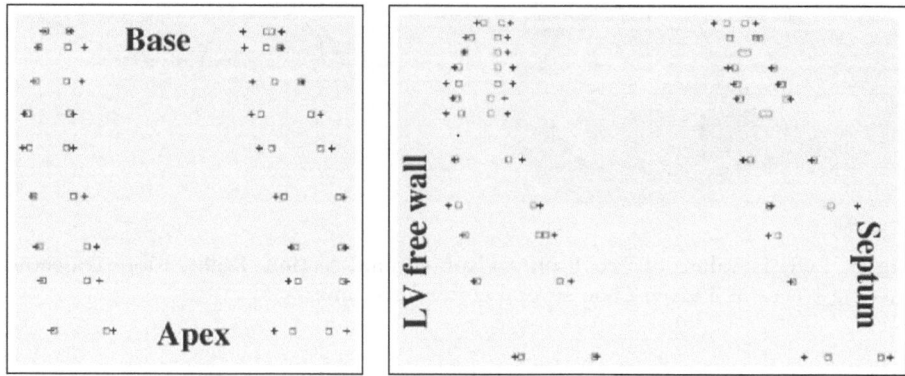

Fig. 4. Traces of some values of C on longitudinal section planes parallel (left) and orthogonal (right) to the interventricular septum.

The conclusion of this study is that checking the invariance of the Clairaut number against experimental values backs up the geodesic conjecture, at least for the left ventricle. In a future work, we intend to study the conjecture for the right ventricle. We will use the fibres tracking algorithm that has already been developed and used for the left ventricle. Simultaneously, an explanation of the geodesic structure in terms of mechanical efficiency will be investigated.

Acknowledgements. This work was supported by the Fonds National de la Science (ACI Modélisation mathématique, mécanique et numérique du myocarde) and by the Région Rhône-Alpes (Projet Mathématiques pour ADéMo).

References

[1] Cai H. (1998) - *Loi de comportement en grandes déformations du muscle à fibres actives. Application à la mécanique du cœur humain et à sa croissance*, Thèse de l'Université de Savoie.

[2] Do Carmo M.P. (1976) - *Differential geometry of curves and surfaces*, Prentice-Hall.

[3] Hutchins G.M. et al (1978) - Shape of the human cardiac ventricles, *Am. J. Cardiol.*, Vol. 41, pp. 646-654.

[4] Jouk P.S., Usson Y., Michalowicz G., and Parazza F. (1995) - Mapping of the orientation of myocardial cells by means of polarized light and confocal scanning laser microscopy, *Microsc. Res. Tech.*, Vol. 30, pp. 480-490.

[5] Jouk P.S., Usson Y., Michalowicz G., and Grossi L. (2000) - Three-dimensional cartography of the pattern of the myofibres in the second trimester fetal human heart, *Anat. Embryol.*, Vol. 202, pp. 103-118.

[6] Hopf H., Rinow W. (1931) - Über den Begriff der vollständigen differentialgeometrischen Flächen, *Comm. Math. Helv.*, Vol. 3, pp. 209-225.

[7] Ohayon J., Usson Y., Jouk P.S., and Cai H. (1998) - Fibre orientation in human fetal heart and ventricular mechanics : A small perturbation analysis, *Comput. Methods Biomechanics Biomedic. Eng.*, Vol. 2, pp. 83-105.

[8] Sanchez-Quintana D., Garcia-Martinez V., Climent V., and Hurle J.M. (1995) - Morphological changes in the normal pattern of ventricular myoarchitecture in the developing human heart, *Anat. Rec.*, Vol. 243, pp. 483-495.

[9] Streeter D.D. (1979) - Gross morphology and fiber geometry of the heart, in *Handbook of Physiology. The cardiovascular system*, Berne R.M., Sperelakis N., Geiger S.R. eds, Am. Phys. Soc., Williams & Wilkins, Baltimore.

Challenges in Modelling
Human Heart's Total Excitation

B. Milan Horáček[1], Kim Simelius[2], Rok Hren[1], and Jukka Nenonen[2]

[1] Dalhousie University, Halifax, Nova Scotia B3H 4H7, Canada,
milan.horacek@dal.ca
[2] Helsinki University of Technology, Laboratory of Biomedical Engineering,
P.O. Box 2200, 02015 HUT, Finland

Abstract. Using a three-dimensional computer model of the human ventricular myocardium, we studied the role of ventricular architecture and conduction system in generating intramural activation patterns and the extracardiac electric field. The model represents the myocardium as an anisotropic bidomain; it incorporates detailed anatomical features, including intramural fiber rotation, the differences in the fiber arrangement of the trabeculae and papillary muscles, and a conduction system. Ectopic activation was elicited at various depths, and "normal" activation was initiated via the conduction system. Extracardiac potentials were calculated throughout each activation sequence. The simulated epicardial potential maps resembled those measured in canine hearts, featuring a central minimum accompanied by two maxima in the early stages of ectopic activation, with the axis joining these extrema approximately parallel to the fibers near the pacing site. The simulated isochrones for the "normal" activation had characteristics very similar to those observed in isolated perfused human hearts.

In the human ventricular myocardium, the anatomical arrangement of intramural fibers [19] and the gross network of interconnecting trabeculae on the endocardial surface, on which are numerous Purkinje strands, create a complex anatomical substrate for the propagation of electrical activity [1]. Both the activation sequence and, perforce, the intracardiac electrograms and/or body-surface electrocardiograms that are associated with it are determined by these anatomical features.

1 Anisotropic Myocardial Structure

The different physical properties observed along the axial and transverse axes of myocardial fibers (anisotropy) are a result of the geometrical arrangement of elongated cells and of the distribution of their gap junctions [21]. When an activation wave front initiated by point stimulation propagates through cardiac muscle, it assumes an ellipsoidal shape that reflects faster conduction along the fibers [5]; the distribution of the potentials generated by the spreading wave front is also affected by the direction of the fibers. Experimental results obtained in

T. Katila et al. (Eds.): FIMH 2001, LNCS 2230, pp. 39–46, 2001.

superfused myocardial laminas [22], on the epicardial and endocardial surfaces of isolated hearts [2], and in a volume conductor surrounding an isolated heart [4] have shown that, in the initial stages of propagation, when activation elicited by point stimulation spreads through fibers that are approximately parallel, potential distributions show a central negative area surrounding the pacing site, accompanied by two positive areas, each with a maximum. The axis joining the two maxima is almost parallel to the fiber direction near the pacing site.

The counterclockwise (CCW) rotation of fibers from epicardium to endo-cardium [19] further affects wave-front shape and associated potential distributions in the later stages of activation. Taccardi et al. [23] recorded, with high spatial resolution, epicardial potential maps from the ventricular surface of exposed canine hearts during ventricular pacing. They identified features of the maps that reveal the direction of the myocardial fibers through which the activation is spreading and investigated how these features vary as a function of pacing site, intramural pacing depth, and post-pacing time. They observed that, during the later phases of propagated activation, the positive areas expand and rotate CCW when the activation wave front propagates from the epicardium to the endocardium, or clockwise (CW) when it propagates from the endocardium to the epicardium; the *asymmetry* of the potential distributions and *multiple maxima* appearing in the expanding positive areas were noted.

Most of these results had been predicted by simulations of Colli Franzone et al. [3] and were substantiated by those of Henriquez et al. [9]. Both of these studies were based on bidomain theory and used a parallelepipedal slab of ventricular tissue with rotational anisotropy. Their simulated activation sequences initiated from epicardial, intramural, and subendocardial sites provided valuable insight into the epicardial and intramural distributions of potentials and activation isochrones, but they were unable to replicate the fragmentation and asymmetry of the expanding and rotating positive areas. Simulating these characteristics would appear to require more realistic models.

Many realistic models have been constructed to simulate propagated activation in the whole heart [8]; among recent models, those introduced by Panfilov [20] and Berenfeld and Jalife [1] are of interest because they incorporate a rotating anisotropy based on meticulously collected canine anatomical data [12,19]. In our previous study [11], we described the effects of the anisotropic structure on epicardial potential distributions in an anatomically realistic model of the *human* ventricular myocardium—based on previously developed propagation algorithm and calculation of extracardiac fields [14,18]—and we tested whether the features that could not be reproduced in idealized models [3,9] can be attributed to the anatomical characteristics of realistic structure. We compared simulated epicardial potentials for paced activation sequences with those recorded [23] during pacing at varying depths in the walls of both ventricles.

Figure 1 shows epicardial maps for activation initiated at pacing sites within the right-ventricular (RV) free wall (5 mm thick, with fibers rotating from $-44°$ at the epicardium to $32°$ at the endocardium). In these distributions, the major axis of the trough in the negative potentials was approximately parallel to the

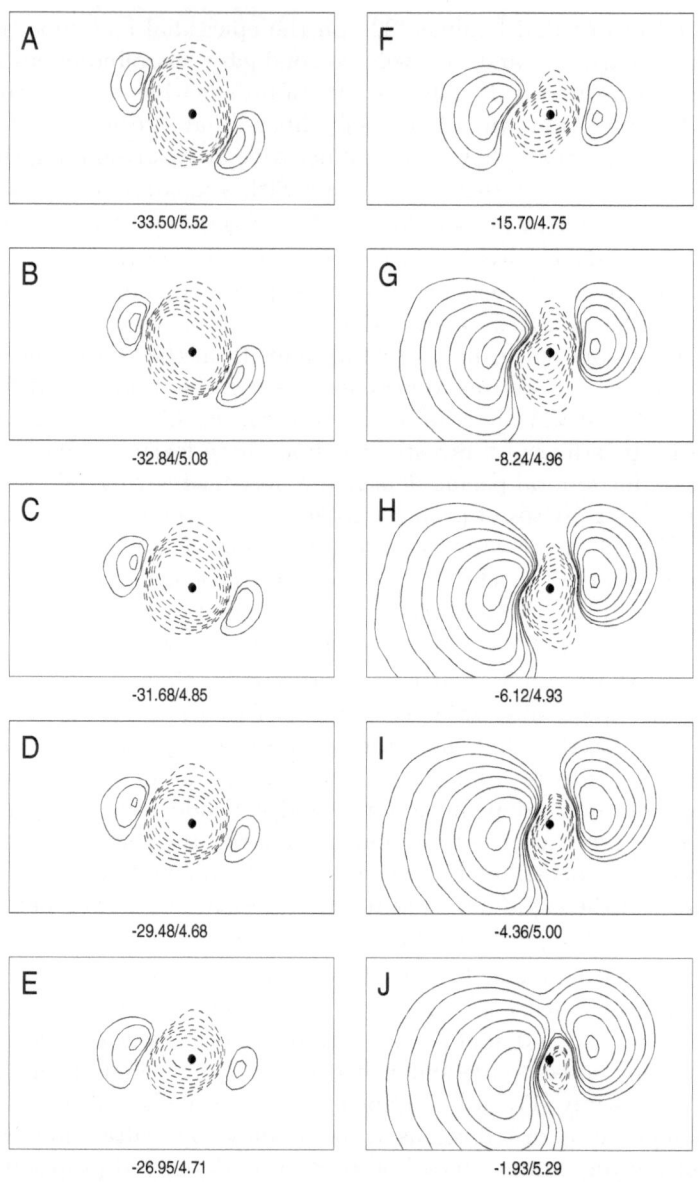

Fig. 1. Simulated epicardial potential maps on a 17×33 grid at 10 ms after the onset of activation for pacing at different intramural depths in the right-ventricular free wall. The pacing sites were 0.5 mm apart, progressing from the epicardium (panel A) to the endocardium (panel J); the epicardial projection of each site is indicated by the filled circle. Isopotential lines are plotted for equal intervals, with no zero line; solid contours represent the positive and broken contours the negative values of potential; the magnitudes of the minimum and maximum are given (in mV) below each map. Note that the axis joining the maxima rotates counterclockwise with increasing pacing depths. From Hren et al. [11], with permission.

local fiber direction at the pacing site, and the positive regions rotated CCW as the pacing depth increased, following the transmural CCW rotation of fibers from the epicardium to the endocardium (Fig. 1B–I). The distance between the maxima did not increase with the pacing depth, unlike in the thicker wall of the left ventricle. The maxima were unequal in strength, with the larger one often on the left side (Fig. 1E–J) of the pacing site.

Depending on the pacing depth, subendocardial and endocardial pacing initially generated epicardial potential distributions that had a single oblong positive area, which developed at 2–18 ms after the onset of activation into the usual pattern with one minimum and two maxima. Distributions calculated at 10 ms after the onset of activation due to an endocardial stimulus at those pacing sites in the right ventricle where the free wall was thinner usually had a central negative area surrounded by a peripheral positive area with two maxima whose joining axis was approximately parallel to the local fiber direction (Fig. 1J). At subendocardial sites in a thick segment of the left-ventricular (LV) free wall with no trabeculae, on the other hand, as the pacing site approached the endocardium, the distance between the maxima decreased, until, for endocardial pacing, a central oblong positive area emerged, from the major axis of which one could clearly deduce the local fiber direction. When the wall also had thick trabeculae, the positive area had no features that one could correlate with the local direction of the fibers. Interestingly, the magnitudes of the maxima did not change monotonically as a function of the pacing depth: they decreased with increased pacing depth until the pacing site approached the endocardium, then started increasing again (Fig. 1). The magnitude of the minimum, on the other hand, usually decreased monotonically with the pacing depth. This agreed with the results from the experimental study [23].

In general, our most important finding is that certain features of measured epicardial potential distributions—such as the fragmentation of the extrema and their asymmetric layout—which could not be reproduced by the slab models [3, 9], can be generated by a realistic model which features a variable wall thickness and recognizes that there are distinct differences in the fiber architecture of compact and trabecular regions of the ventricular wall.

2   Specialized Conduction System

Knowledge of the anatomy and distribution of the human atrioventricular (A-V) conduction system is important in understanding the sequence of "normal" ventricular activation and in establishing the anatomical basis of conduction disorders. The A-V conduction system begins at the A-V node and the bundle of His, proceeds through an area of fibrous tissue on top of the interventricular septum, and divides into the left and right bundle branches [6,17], which ramify subendocardially throughout the left and right ventricles into the Purkinje plexus. Fibers that fit the anatomical description of Purkinje fibers and show action potentials similar to those seen in the bundle of His are found throughout

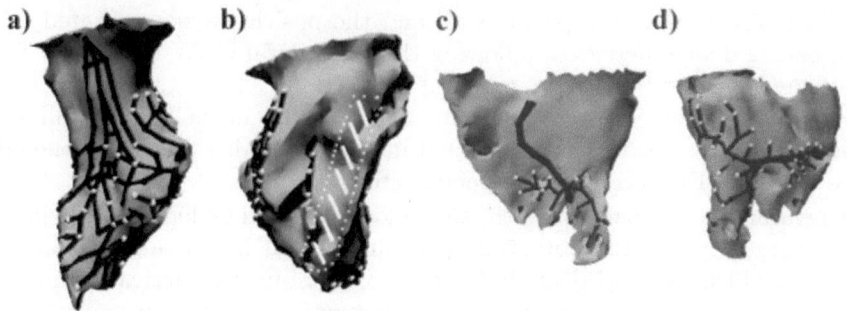

Fig. 2. The geometry of the modelled conduction system in different views. The views of the LV septum (a) and LV free wall (b) show the complex structure stemming from the left bundle branch; note the vertical spiral gap (dashed area) in the LV conduction system in (b). The right bundle branch is shown on the RV septum (c) and the RV free wall (d). The Purkinje-myocardial junctions, at which the conduction system connects with the ventricular myocardium, are shown as light circles.

the bundle branches, in false tendons [16], in an endocardial mesh, and in the *chordae tendinae* [10].

The anatomy of the left bundle branch (LBB) is extremely variable [25]. The LBB has usually been found to be initially a sheet-like structure, which then splits into three separate divisions with multiple interconnections [6], then it fans out over the LV septal surface [17] and its divisions extend towards the bases of anterior and posterior papillary muscles, while the posterior rim is oriented towards the LV posterior papillary muscle. The right bundle branch (RBB) usually begins from the most distal part of the bundle of His [25], crosses over to the RV through fibrous tissue on top of the muscular interventricular septum, courses just beneath the endocardial surface of the RV septum before it emerges near the base of the RV anterior papillary muscle; from there it branches into fascicles leading to the posterior papillary muscle and the RV free wall. In the human heart, there is no evidence of penetration of the Purkinje fibers intramurally, as has been observed in other species [26]. From the Purkinje plexus, activation is conveyed to the myocardium by transitional cells in Purkinje-myocardial junctions (PMJs) [1,26].

We have developed software for the interactive editing of the conduction system in our model of the ventricular myocardium. The user can create nodes on the endocardial surface by pointing to the desired locations, and connect them as required. These nodes can later be repositioned, and the connections can be either retained or modified. Some nodes are just bifurcation points for the conduction system; some are PMJs. The thickness of the connections and the extent of the PMJ patches are adjustable, to ensure connectivity and proper propagation between the conduction system and the myocardium. The propagation velocity in the conduction system was set to approximately 2.0 m/s.

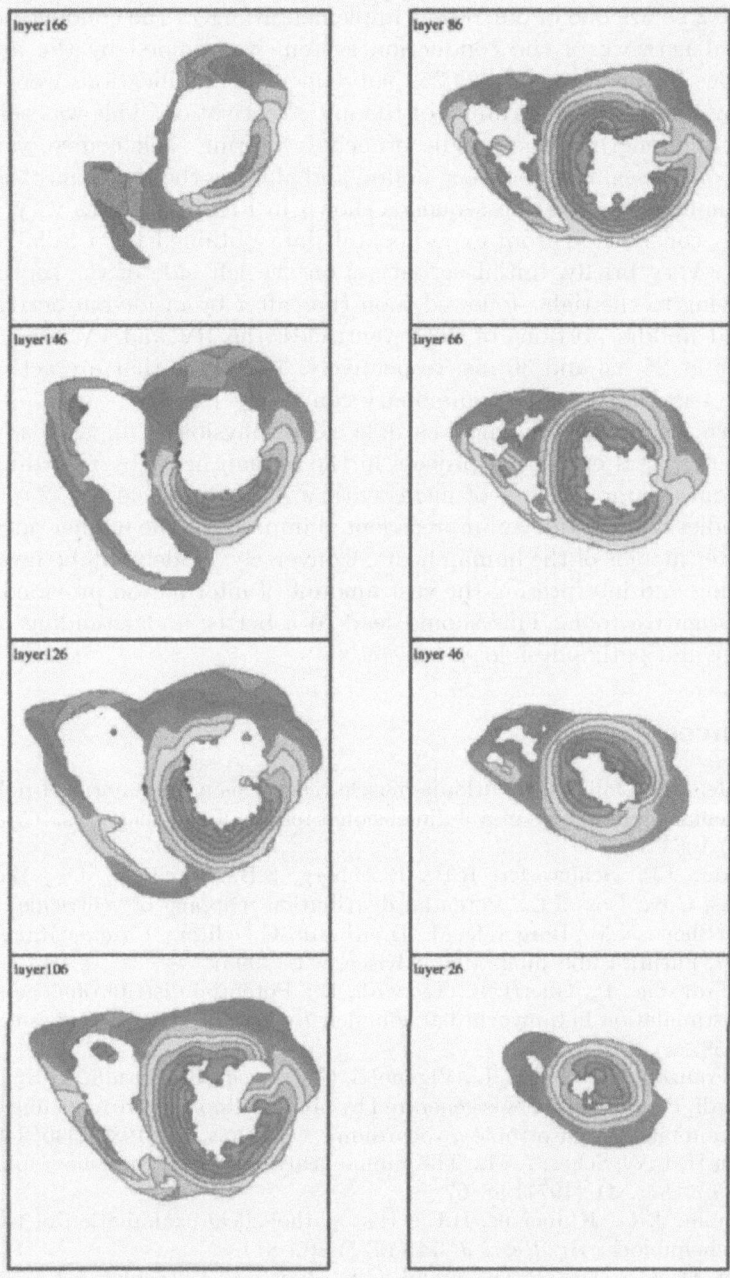

Fig. 3. Simulated isochrones of activation in a three-dimensional computer model of the human ventricular myocardium. The horizonal layers—numbered 166, ... , 26, from base to apex—correspond to sections depicted by Durrer et al. [7]; each color represents a 5-ms interval, and the color coding of the activation times is the same as in [7] (except we use black to indicate the first 5 ms of activation in the conduction system).

Figure 2 shows one of our recent implementations of the conduction system. The initial network of the conduction system was guided by the anatomical descriptions in the literature [24,25]; subsequently, modifications were made interactively, to balance the timing of the initial activation. This was achieved by adjusting the length of the bundle branches, altering their course, varying the thickness of the segments between nodes, and altering the locations of the PMJs.

The simulated activation sequence shown in Figure 3 agrees very well with isochrones constructed from experimental data obtained from isolated human hearts [7]. Very briefly, initial activity is on the left side of the septum (layer 106), moving to the right, followed soon thereafter by inside-out activity in the apical and middle portions of both ventricles; the RV and LV breakthroughs take place at 25 ms and 30 ms, respectively. The areas that are activated last are in the basal RV near the pulmonary conus (layer 166).

Modern techniques of clinical cardiac electrophysiology allow *in situ* investigation of the total excitation process in the human heart by recording electric signals from a large number of intracavitary [13] or endocardial [2] electrodes. These studies will provide an unprecedented impetus to the further development of computer models of the human heart. Conversely, models will be invaluable in synthesizing and interpreting the vast amount of information provided by these new investigative tools. This should lead to a better understanding of cardiac physiology and pathophysiology.

References

1. Berenfeld, O., Jalife, J.: Purkinje-muscle reentry as a mechanism of polymorphic ventricular arrhythmias in a 3-dimensional model of the ventricles. *Circ. Res.* **82** (1998) 1063–1077
2. Boineau, J.P., Schluessler, R.B., Eisenberg, S.B., Tweddell, J.S., Harada, A., Rokkas, C.K., Cox, J.L.: Potential distribution mapping of ventricular tachycardia. In Shenasa, M., Borggrefe, M., Breithardt, G., editors, *Cardiac Mapping*, pages 85–107. Futura Publishing, Mount Kisco, NY (1993)
3. Colli Franzone, P., Guerri, L., Taccardi, B.: Potential distributions generated by point stimulation in a myocardial volume. *J. Cardiovasc. Electrophysiol.* **4** (1993) 438–458
4. Colli Franzone, P., Guerri, L., Viganotti, C., Macchi, E., Baruffi, S., Spaggiari, S., Taccardi, B.: Potential fields generated by oblique dipole layers modeling excitation wavefronts in the anisotropic myocardium. *Circ. Res.* **51** (1982) 330–346
5. Corbin II, L.V., Scher, A.M.: The canine heart as an electrocardiographic generator. *Circ. Res.* **41** (1977) 58–67
6. Demoulin, J.-C., Kulbertus, H.E.: Histopathological examination of the concept of left hemiblock. *Br. Heart J.* **34** (1972) 807–814
7. Durrer, D., van Dam, R.Th., Freud, G.E., Janse, M.J., Meijler, F.L., Arzbaecher, R.C.: Total excitation of the isolated human heart. *Circulation* **41** (1970) 899–912
8. Gulrajani, R.M.: Models of the electrical activity of the heart and the computer simulation of the electrocardiogram. *CRC Crit. Rev. Biomed. Eng.* **16** (1988) 1–66
9. Henriquez, C.S., Muzikant, A.L., Smoak, C.K.: Anisotropy, fiber curvature and bath loading effects on activation in thin and thick cardiac tissue preparations. *J. Cardiovasc. Electrophysiol.* **7** (1996) 424–444

10. Hoffman, B.F., Cranefield, P.F.: *Electrophysiology of the heart*. McGraw-Hill, New York, NY (1960)
11. Hren, R., Nenonen, J., Horáček, B.M.: Simulated epicardial potential maps during paced activation reflect myocardial fibrous structure. *Ann. Biomed. Eng.* **26** (1998) 1022–1035
12. Hunter, P.J., Smaill, B.H., Nielsen, P.M.F., LeGrice, I.J.: A mathematical model of cardiac anatomy. In Panfilov, A.V., Holden, A.V., editors, *Computational Biology of the Heart*, pages 171–215. Wiley, New York (1997)
13. Khoury, D.S., Taccardi, B., Lux, R.L., Ershler, P.R., Rudy, Y.: Reconstruction of endocardial potentials and activation sequences from intracavitary probe measurements. *Circulation* **91** (1995) 845–863
14. Leon, L.J., Horáček, B.M.: Computer model of excitation and recovery in the anisotropic myocardium. *J. Electrocardiol.* **24** (1991) 1–41
15. Lewis, T.: *The mechanism and graphic registration of the heart beat*. Shaw & Sons, London (1925) 3rd Edition.
16. Luetmer, P.H., Edwards, W.D., Seward, J.B., Tajik, J.: Incidence and distribution of left ventricular false tendons. *J. Am. Coll. Cardiol.* **8** (1986) 179–183
17. Massing, G.K., James, T.N.: Anatomical configuration of the His bundle and bundle branches in the human heart. *Circulation* **53** (1976) 609–621
18. Nenonen, J., Edens, J.A., Leon, L.J., Horáček, B.M.: Computer model of propagated excitation in the anisotropic human heart. I. Implementation and algorithms. II. Simulation of extracardiac fields. In Murray, A., Arzbäecher, R., editors, *Computers in Cardiology*, pages 545–548 and 217–220. IEEE Computer Society Press, Los Alamitos, CA (1991)
19. Nielsen, P.M.F., LeGrice, I.J., Smaill, B.H., Hunter, P.J.: Mathematical model of geometry and fibrous structure of the heart. *Am. J. Physiol.* **260** (1991) H1365–H1378
20. Panfilov, A.V.: Modelling of re-entrant patterns in an anatomical model of the heart. In Panfilov, A.V., Holden, A.V., editors, *Computational Biology of the Heart*, pages 259–276. Wiley, New York (1997)
21. Spach, M.S.: Anisotropy of cardiac tissue: A major determinant of conduction? *J. Cardiovasc. Electrophysiol.* **10** (1999) 887–890
22. Spach, M.S., Miller III, W.T., Miller-Jones, E., Warren, R.B., Barr, R.C.: Extracellular potentials related to intracellular action potentials during impulse conduction in anisotropic canine cardiac muscle. *Circ. Res.* **45** (1979) 188–204
23. Taccardi, B., Macchi, E., Lux, R.L., Ershler, P.E., Spaggiari, S., Baruffi, S., Vyhmeister, Y.: Effect of myocardial fiber direction on epicardial potentials. *Circulation* **90** (1994) 3076–3090
24. Tawara, S.: *The conduction system of the mammalian heart. An anatomico-histological study of the atrioventricular bundle and the Purkinje fibres*. Imperial College Press, London (2000)
25. Titus, J.L.: Normal anatomy of the human cardiac conduction system. *Mayo Clinic Proc.* **48** (1973) 24–30
26. Tranum-Jensen, J., Wilde, A.A.M., Vermeulen, J.T., Janse, M.J.: Morphology of electrophysiologically identified junctions between Purkinje fibers and ventricular muscle in rabbit and pig hearts. *Circ. Res.* **69** (1991) 429–437

Two-Dimensional Ultrasonic Strain Rate Measurement of the Human Heart in Vivo

Jan D'hooge[1], Fadi Jamal[2], Bart Bijnens[2], Jan Thoen[3], Frans Van de Werf[2], George R. Sutherland[2], and Paul Suetens[1]

[1] Medical Image Computing, Department of Electrical Engineering, Catholic University of Leuven, Leuven, Belgium
jan.dhooge@uz.kuleuven.ac.be,
http://www.medicalimagecomputing.be
[2] Department of Cardiology, Catholic University of Leuven, Leuven, Belgium
[3] Laboratorium voor akoestiek en thermische fysica, Department of physics, Catholic University of Leuven, Leuven, Belgium

Abstract. In this study, the feasibility of two-dimensional strain rate estimation of the human heart in vivo is shown. To do this, ultrasonic B-mode data were captured at a high temporal resolution of 3.7 ms and processed off-line. The motion of the radio-frequency signal patterns within the two-dimensional sector image was tracked and used as the basis for strain rate estimation. Both axial and lateral motion and strain rate estimates showed a good agreement with the results obtained by more established, one-dimensional techniques.

1 Introduction

Regional strain and strain rate imaging have been introduced as new clinical tools to quantify regional myocardial function [1]. The most widely used method for cardiac strain rate estimation is based on myocardial velocity imaging, i.e. Doppler myocardial imaging [2]. This methodology has been validated both in vitro [3] and in vivo [4] and has been shown to be clinically applicable both in the experimental and clinical settings. However, a major drawback of the existing approaches is that they are limited to making only a one-dimensional measurement. Indeed, only the strain (rate) along an image line can be assessed. This limitation causes the technique to be angle dependent [5]. As a result, current ultrasound-based cardiac deformation data sets are incomplete. This could limit their application in quantifying cardiac function.

In the field of ultrasound elastography other approaches to strain estimation by ultrasound have been described [6,7]. Some of these were shown to allow two-dimensional strain estimation by the tracking of radio frequency (RF) patterns within a two-dimensional RF image [8]. The purpose of this study was to test the applicability of such techniques to the heart and to make a multi-dimensional measurement of myocardial strain (rate) in vivo.

T. Katila et al. (Eds.): FIMH 2001, LNCS 2230, pp. 47–52, 2001.
© Springer-Verlag Berlin Heidelberg 2001

2 Methods

2.1 Data Acquisition

Cardiac ultrasound data were acquired from a young, healthy volunteer using an ultrasound scanner (GE Vingmed, System V, Horten, Norway) which allowed the continuous acquisition of digital IQ data (In-phase Quadrature sampled RF data [9]). A dedicated pulse sequence was developed in order to obtain B-mode data sets with high temporal resolution. To do this, the scan angle was reduced to 10 degrees and the number of RF image lines was set at 12. This resulted in an effective RF acquisition rate of 270 Hz.

During apnea, a complete cardiac cycle of ultrasound data from the interventricular septum was acquired in an apical four chamber view using this dedicated pulse sequence. A standard 2.5 MHz phased array transducer (FPA 2.5MHz 1C) was used for fundamental imaging. Finally, the data acquired were transfered to a workstation for further off-line processing.

2.2 Strain Rate Estimation

RF data were reconstructed from the IQ data set. After axial and lateral linear interpolation of the RF data set (by a factor 2 and 8 respectively, resulting in spatial sampling of approximately 20 and 150 μm in the axial and lateral directions at the maximal image depth), the motion of the RF patterns between two successive RF frames was estimated using a newly developed algorithm which was based on the methodology described by previous authors [8]. However, in order to determine the time lag between two signal windows, the Sum of Absolute Differences (SAD) function [10] rather than the cross-correlation function was used. Moreover, temporal stretching (range : 0.97–1.03) of the first signal window, as presented in [11], showed to be indispensable. Window lengths were chosen to be 64 and 192 (interpolated) samples (corresponding to 1.2 and 3.7 mm) for the pattern to be tracked and the search region respectively. A window overlap of 50% was used and the lateral search range was set to 17 (interpolated) image lines.

The axial and lateral strains between two subsequent images were calculated as the axial and lateral spatial gradients of the axial and lateral motion estimates respectively [8]. Prior to applying a gradient operator, the axial motion estimates were median filtered (five pixels) to remove outliers and the lateral motion estimates were low-pass filtered by convolving them with a rectangular window of eleven pixels length. The gradient operator consisted of a linear fit through eleven consecutive motion estimates. Finally, the extracted strain values were normalized by the frame rate in order to obtain the axial and lateral strain rates respectively.

3 Results

Figure 1 (a) shows a M-mode image and an individual profile at a depth of 7 cm of the axial strain rate estimates over one R-R interval. The cycle starts with a short period of negative strain rate which is followed by a longer period of muscle shortening, which ends approximately 260 ms after the onset of cardiac contraction. During the next 80 ms, strain rate values of different sign are found for the apical and basal regions. Subsequently, a bi-phasic lengthening is measured, separated by a period in which length remains constant. The axial strain rates are homogeneous throughout the cardiac wall.

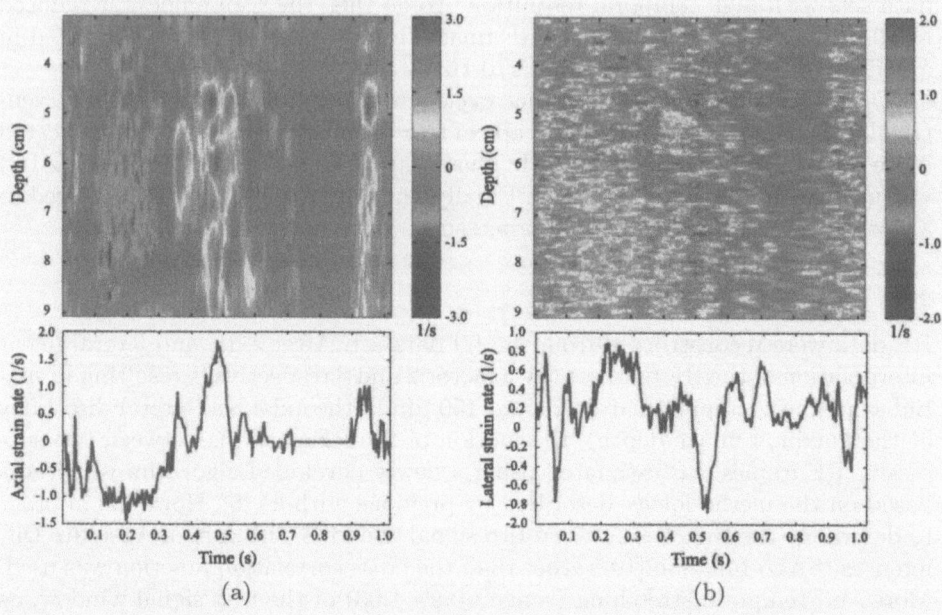

Fig. 1. M-mode image and an individual profile of the axial (a) and lateral (b) strain rate estimates of the interventricular septum. The profiles were extracted at a depth of 7 cm.

The same images are presented for the lateral strain rate estimates in figure 1 (b). The lateral strain rate estimates are noisier than the axial ones but positive strain rates during the first 260 ms of the cardiac cycle can be observed. After this, a period of positive and negative lateral strain rates occur in the basal and apical regions respectively. Approximately 350 ms after the onset of the cardiac cycle, negative strain rates are measured throughout the cardiac wall. These are followed by a period of zero strain rate. Finally, another period of deformation is observed during the last 100 ms of the cardiac cycle.

4   Discussion

The strain rate patterns in normal individuals, derived by tissue Doppler methods, have been described extensively [1,12,13]. The longitudinal strain rate of the septal wall, as assessed from the apical four chamber view, is negative during systole (representing shortening of the muscle) and shows a bi-phasic lengthening (positive strain rates) during diastole. The first diastolic lengthening phase is caused by a combination of relaxation of the cardiac muscle and early filling, while the second is a result of the increasing intraventricular pressure following filling due to atrial contraction. Both lengthening phases are separated by a period of constant length which corresponds to cardiac diastasis. It has been observed that isovolumetric contraction and relaxation are accompanied by a rapid change in shape of the ventricle [14]. This results in a significant amount of out-of-plane motion. Rapid changes in myocardial motion and strain rate estimates have been reported during these periods. The average peak longitudinal strain rate values reported for systole, early and late diastolic filling are respectively : -1.5, 2.0 and 1.0 s^{-1} [13]. These have been shown to be homogeneous throughout the septum.

To date, radial strain rates in the septum have not been studied by an appropriate method as current tissue Doppler methodology does not allow this. Indeed, radial strain rates can only be assessed from a parasternal transducer position. Using this approach, the septum is usually located in the near field of the probe. However, the radial strain rate of the posterior wall has been measured accurately and it seems fair to assume that the septal wall shows a similar behavior : systolic thickening (positive strain rates) and bi-phasic diastolic thinning (negative strain rates).

All of the regional strain rate characteristics already described in the literature can be seen in figure 1 (a) and (b). In the apical four chamber view, the axial and lateral strain rate estimates correspond to the longitudinal and radial strain rates respectively [2]. Axial estimates were homogeneous throughout the septal wall; they showed shortening during systole and bi-phasic lengthening during diastole. Moreover, it can be observed that longitudinal deformation of the septal wall during atrial filling starts at the base and moves towards the apex. This phenomenon has well been described both in strain rate studies of the normal left ventricle and in computer simulations of left ventricular filling [15,16]. It is most likely the result of the propagation of a pressure wave and its associated blood vortex that enter the left ventricle through the mitral valve during atrial filling [15,16]. The radial strain rate estimates are noisier but the different phases of the cardiac cycle can still be identified : systolic thickening of the muscle followed by a bi-phasic diastolic phase. Both axial and lateral strain rate estimates had an isovolumetric relaxation time around 80 ms. This corresponds to the normal values in the literature [17].

Although our results demonstrate the feasibility of in vivo, two-dimensional myocardial strain rate estimation by means of RF tracking, much can be improved. Firstly, in order to construct the images presented in this report, no attempt was made to track the underlying tissue. This implies that the strain rate profiles shown, may contain information derived from differing anatomic regions. Nevertheless, the different phases of the cardiac cycle were distinguished.

Secondly, the lateral gradient operator was applied on all lateral motion estimates. As the outermost image lines were taken from the blood pool, this means
that a possible source of noise in the lateral motion estimates was introduced.
However, avoiding this effect requires more complex post-processing as the septal wall moves laterally in the image during the cardiac cycle. Note that this
lateral motion was clearly detected by the lateral motion estimator. This is one
of the major advantages of this methodology : two-dimensional velocities, displacements, strain rates and strains can be extracted simultaneously. Finally, as
the RF images were taken in a sector format, image lines diverge with depth.
This implies that the intrinsic accuracy and noise characteristics of the lateral
estimates will be depth dependent. Moreover, parameters such as line density,
frame rate and interleaving will have a marked influence on the quality of the
lateral motion and strain rate estimates. Tackling these problems in order to
improve these two-dimensional estimates is left for future work.

5 Conclusions

In this paper the feasibility of two-dimensional strain rate estimation of the
human heart in vivo was shown. Hereto, RF data sets of high temporal resolution
were acquired and subsequently processed to extract motion and strain rate
estimates based on a RF tracking algorithm. The properties of the extracted
axial and lateral estimates showed a good correspondence to results found in the
literature. Although many aspects could be improved, these initial results show
that multi-dimensional myocardial strain rate estimation in vivo is feasible.

Acknowledgments. This work was supported by the Fund for Scientific Research – Flanders (FWO). The authors would like to thank GE Vingmed for
their technical assistance of the project.

References

1. A. Heimdal, A. Stoylen, H. Torp, and T. Skjaerpe. Real-time strain rate imaging
   of the left ventricle by ultrasound. *Journal of the American Society of Echocardiography*, 11(11):1013–1019, 1998.
2. J. D'hooge, A. Heimdal, F. Jamal, T. Kukulski, B. Bijnens, F. Rademakers, L. Hatle, P. Suetens, and G.R. Sutherland. Regional strain and strain rate measurements
   by cardiac ultrasound: principles, implementation and limitations. *European Journal of Echocardiography*, 1(3):154–170, 2000.
3. A. Heimdal, J. D'hooge, B. Bijnens, G.R. Sutherland, and H. Torp. In vitro validation of in-plane strain rate imaging. a new ultrasound technique for evaluating regional myocardial deformation based on tissue doppler imaging. (abstract).
   Echocardiography, 18(8):S40, 1998.
4. S. Urheim, T. Edvardsen, H. Torp, B. Angelsen, and O. Smiseth. Myocardial strain
   by doppler echocardiography. validation of a new method to quantify regional
   myocardial function. *Circulation*, 102:1158–1164, 2000.

52   J. D'hooge et al.

5. P.L. Castro, N.L. Greenberg, J. Drinko, M.J. Garcia, and J.D. Thomas. Potential pitfalls of strain rate imaging: angle dependency. *Biomedical sciences instrumentation*, 36:197–202, 2000.
6. I.A. Hein and W.D. O'Brien. Current time domain methods for assessing tissue motion by analysis from reflected ultrasound echoes – a review. *IEEE Transactions on Ultrasonics, Ferro-electrics and Frequency Control*, 40(2):84–102, 1993.
7. L. Gao, K.J. Parker, R.M. Lerner, and S.F. Levinson. Imaging of the elastic properties of tissue – a review. *Ultrasound in Medicine & Biology*, 22(8):959–977, 1996.
8. E.E. Konofagou and J. Ophir. A new method for estimation and imaging of lateral strains and poisson's ratios in tissues. *Ultrasound in Medicine & Biology*, 24:1183–1199, 1998.
9. J.G. Proakis and D.G. Manolakis. *Digital signal processing: principles, algorithms and applications*. Prentice-Hall International, 1996.
10. L.N. Bohs and G.E. Trahey. A novel method for angle independent ultrasonic imaging of blood flow and tissue motion. *IEEE Transactions on Biomedical Engineering*, 38:280–286, 1991.
11. T. Varghese, J. Ophir, and I. Cespedes. Noise reduction in elastography using temporal stretching with multicompression averaging. *Ultrasound in Medicine & Biology*, 22:1042–1053, 1996.
12. J.U. Voigt, M.F. Arnold, M. Karlsson, L. Hubbert, T. Kukulski, L. Hatle, and G.R. Sutherland. Assessment of regional longitudinal myocardial strain rate derived from doppler myocardial imaging indexes in normal and infarcted myocardium. *The Journal of the American Society of Echocardiography*, 13(6):588–598, 2000.
13. M. Kowalski, T. Kukulski, F. Jamal, J. D'hooge, F. Weidemann, F. Rademakers, B. Bijnens, L. Hatle, and G.R. Sutherland. Can natural strain and strain rate quantify regional myocardial deformation? a study in healthy subjects. *Ultrasound in Medicine & Biology*, 27(8):1087–1097, 2001.
14. F.E. Rademakers, M.B. Buchalter, W.J. Rogers, E.A. Zerhouni, J.L. Weisfeldt, M.L. Weiss, and B. Shapiro. Dissociation between left ventricular untwisting and filling. accentuation by catecholamines. *Circulation*, 85(4):1572–1581, 1992.
15. J.A. Vierendeels, K. Riemslagh, E. Dick, and P.R. Verdonck. Computer simulation of intraventricular flow and pressure gradients during diastole. *Journal of Biomechanical Engineering*, 122(6):667–674, 2000.
16. J.U. Voigt, G. Lindenmeier, D. Werner, F.A. Flachskampf, U. Nixdorff, L. Hatle, G.R. Sutherland, and W.G. Daniel. Strain rate imaging for the assessment of preload dependent changes in regional left ventricular diastolic longitudinal function. *Journal of the American Society of Echocardiography*, page (In Press), 2001.
17. C.P. Appleton and L. Hatle. The natural history of left ventricular filling abnormalities: assessment by two-dimensional and doppler echocardiography. *Echocardiography*, 9:437–457, 1992.

Deformation Field Estimation for the Cardiac Wall Using Doppler Tissue Imaging

Valérie Moreau[1], Laurent D. Cohen[1], and Denis Pellerin[2]

[1] CEREMADE, University of Paris-Dauphine, 75775 Paris cedex 16, France,
{moreau,cohen}@ceremade.dauphine.fr
[2] St George's Hospital Medical School, University of London

Abstract. This paper presents different ways to use the Doppler Tissue Imaging (DTI) in order to determine deformation of the cardiac wall. As an extra information added to the ultrasound images, the DTI gives the velocity in the direction of the sensor. We first show a way to track points along the cardiac wall in a M-Mode image (1D+t). This is based on energy minimization similar to a deformable grid. We then extend the ideas to finding the deformation field in a sequence of 2D images (2D+t). This is based on energy minimization including spatio-temporal regularization and a priori constraints.

Keywords: Cardiac image processing, Ultrasound Image, Doppler Tissue Imaging, motion estimation, multi-modality image fusion.

1 Introduction

Doppler Tissue Imaging (DTI) is a recent technique which provides a partial information about the myocardial wall velocities. This is the velocity of the tissues in the direction of the sensor. This new data is represented by a colour added to the conventional ultrasound image. Two types of these images are used by the cardiologists. First 2D images as in figure 1.a. are usually employed in ultrasound imaging. But the extra data which is collected during the acquisition implies a reduction of the temporal resolution compared to classical ultrasound. We cannot have more than a hundred images per second. M-Mode images (Figure 1.b) can give a better temporal resolution by reducing the studied area. They are obtained by choosing a 1D segment on the image and watching its evolution through time. Since there is only one dimension the temporal resolution is increased to about 500 frames per second. In this work, we used sequences of images of left ventricle of human hearts.

Previously, M-mode images have been studied in [1] in order to track the cardiac wall with a variant of active contours. The contour $C(t) = (t, f(t))$ deforms to minimize $E(f) = \int_0^T \omega_1 |f'(t)|^2 + \omega_2 |f''(t)|^2 + P_{edge}(C(t)) + P_{velocity}(C(t))dt$. P_{edge} and $P_{velocity}$ are potentials which attract respectively $C(t)$ to the edge and $f'(t)$ close to the velocity measured by the DTI. [1] shows the advantage of using DTI in addition to the edge information.

We will use different variational methods to study the deformation of the heart in M-mode and afterwards 2D DTI images.

T. Katila et al. (Eds.): FIMH 2001, LNCS 2230, pp. 53–60, 2001.

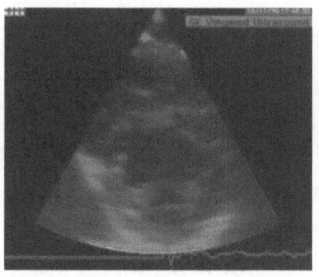 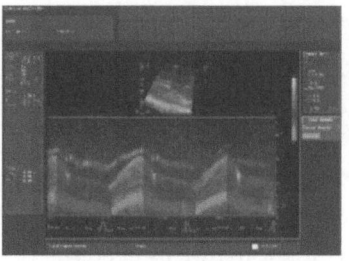

(a) 2D Ultrasound Image.   (b) M-Mode Ultrasound Image.

Fig. 1. DTI Images.

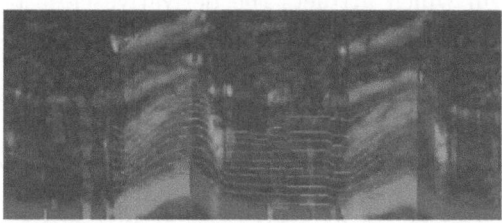

Fig. 2. Initialization of the steepest gradient descent.

2 Tracking the Wall through M-Mode Images

We now want to track several points through the cardiac wall on the M-Mode image $I(t,z)$, making use of the velocity given by the DTI image $v_{DTI}(t,z)$. Points are chosen for the initial time $t = 0$ along a hand given segment. They are regularly spaced on this vertical segment as seen on the left of figure 2.

Let $\{C_i(t) = (t, y_i(t))\}_{1 \leq i \leq N}$ be the curves which perform the tracking of these points. If the points we want to follow are close enough, the curves $\{C_1, \ldots, C_N\}$ must be consistent with one another. In order to improve the tracking, we will consider the set of curves $\{C_1, \ldots, C_N\}$ as an active net: $(y(t,s) = y_s(t))_{s,t}$ where only the second coordinate $y(t,s)$ can vary. The active nets, or deformable grids, are defined in [2] and [3]. The net deforms according to the minimization of an energy. Our energy consists of three terms.

1. A regularization term as in [2].
   $$E_{reg}(y) = \iint \alpha(\tfrac{\partial y}{\partial s}^2 + \tfrac{\partial y}{\partial t}^2) + \beta(\tfrac{\partial^2 y}{\partial s^2}^2 + 2\tfrac{\partial^2 y}{\partial st}^2 + \tfrac{\partial^2 y}{\partial t^2}^2)dtds$$
   This term will be the one enabling interaction between successive curves. The first derivatives make the net contracts (which should be avoided by choosing α small) and the second derivatives enforce smoothness and rigidity.

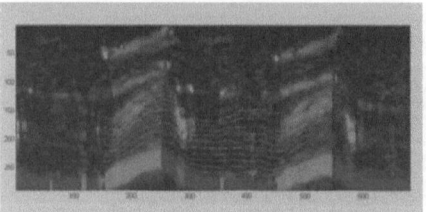 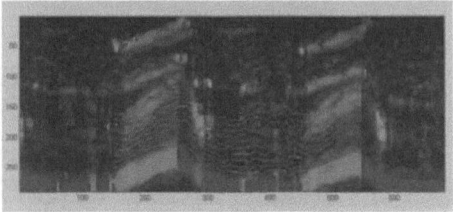

(a) After a few iterations of steep-   (b) Result of the tracking.
est gradient descent.

Fig. 3. Steepest gradient descent.

2. An external term which attracts the derivative close to the given velocity
   measured by the DTI. This is an extension in two dimensions of [1].
   $E_{velocity}(y) = \int\int (\frac{\partial y}{\partial t} - v_{DTI}(t, y(t, s)))^2 dtds$
3. The last term is also an external term. We assume that the gray level is nearly
   constant along and around each curve.
   $E_{gray}(y) = \int\int \sum_{k=-2}^{k=2} (I(t, y(t, s) + k) - I(0, y(0, s) + k)^2 dsdt$

We used both DTI and gray scale conventional ultrasound in this energy.
The net y is obtained by the minimization of $E(y) = E_{reg}(y) + \mu E_{gray}(y) + \lambda E_{velocity}(y)$ where λ and μ are postive constants. μ must be chosen small because E_{gray} is very sensitive to noise. We proceed as in [1] and [4] and use a
steepest gradient descent, the discretization was done by finite differences. This
gives in matrix form $(Id + \tau A)Y^{n+1} = Y^n + \tau F(Y^n)$ where Y is the discrete
version of y and A is a sparse square matrix. To avoid a large matrix inversion,
we can approximate $(Id + \tau A)^{-1} \approx Id - \tau A$ for τ small enough. We then apply a
SOR algorithm [5]. The energy can have many local minima. Therefore we must

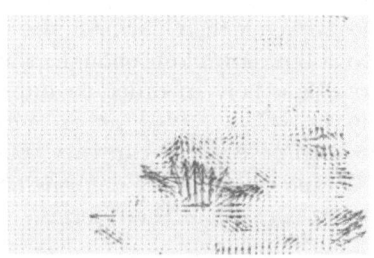 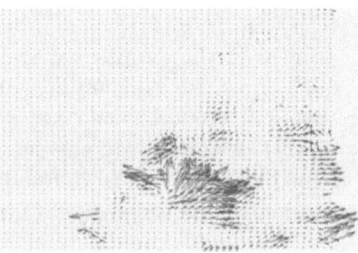

(a) Optical Flow. Close up.   (b) Velocity field obtained by
Bottom of the lateral wall.   our method on the same case.

Fig. 4. Comparison between optical flow and the velocity field we obtained. In these
images, the sensor is above and on the right of the pictures.

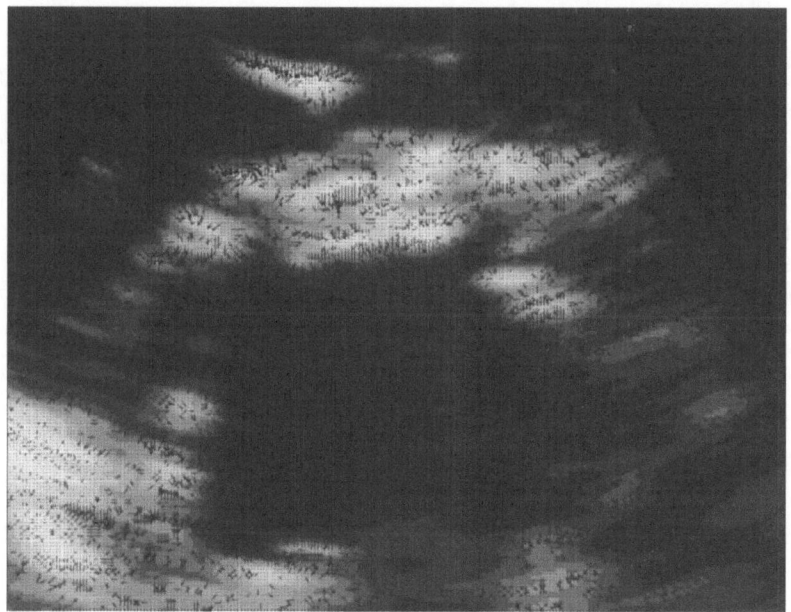

Fig. 5. Velocity field with the simplest method.

use an initialization close to the solution. For this purpose, we choose an integration of the velocity measured by the DTI: $y(t+1,s) \approx y(t,s) + v_{DTI}(t,y(t,s))dt$ (figure 2) where dt is the time step. These curves, which are the direct interpretation of the DTI velocity do not provide an accurate tracking of the wall. We can see that some curves leave the wall during the tracking. The hypothesis about the gray level is not exact in the case of ultrasound images. Nevertheless figure 3 shows how this term of the energy tends to correct the tracking processed using only DTI. Figure 3.b presents a final result. We have compared these curves to manually traced curves by the cardiologist. We notice that the set of curves folow precisely the deformation of the cardiac wall. This automatic tracking has been of much help for cardiolgists in order to study various use of DTI images [6], [7].

3   Deformation Field in a 2D Image Sequence

3.1   Presentation

Our next interest is the study of 2D image sequences. The difficulties raised are the low temporal resolution and the incomplete DTI information. The DTI only measures the velocity in the direction of the sensor. Moreover the acquisition of the sequence instead of a single image implies a lower spatial resolution. Our motivation is to be able to diagnose a pathology with the help of DTI ultrasound images. For that purpose, we are mostly interested in recovering a complete deformation field.

3.2 Recovering the Velocity Field

The DTI sequence contains two types of information: the velocity $v_{DTI}(x, y, t)$ in the direction of the sensor measured by the DTI and the conventional ultrasound sequence $I(x, y, t)$. We will use this second information to complete the first one. From the grayscale conventional ultrasound sequence, we can calculate the optical flow [8], [11], [9] and [10]. The optical flow is the distribution of apparent velocity of motion of brightness patterns in an image. The determination of the optical flow is based on the hypothesis that the brightness of a point $I(x(t), y(t), t)$ is constant through time. Using the chain rule for differentiation we see that $\frac{\partial I}{\partial x}\frac{\partial x}{\partial t} + \frac{\partial I}{\partial y}\frac{\partial y}{\partial t} + \frac{\partial I}{\partial t} = 0$. If we let $u = \frac{\partial x}{\partial t}$ and $v = \frac{\partial y}{\partial t}$, we have a linear equation in the two unknows u and $v : I_x u + I_y v + I_t = 0$, where $I_x = \frac{\partial I}{\partial x}$,

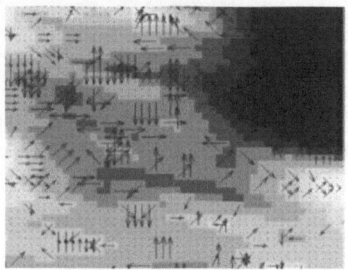

Fig. 6. Close up on figure 5.

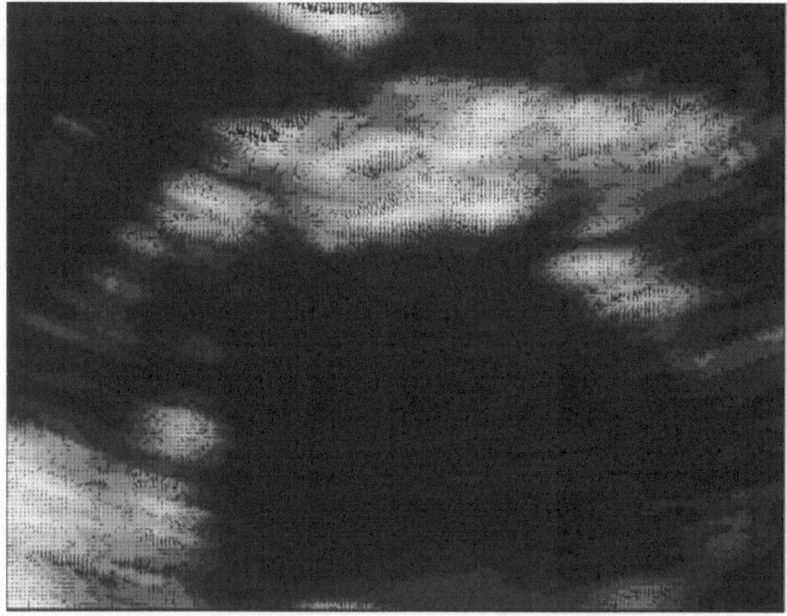

Fig. 7. Velocity field with a spatio-temporal regularization.

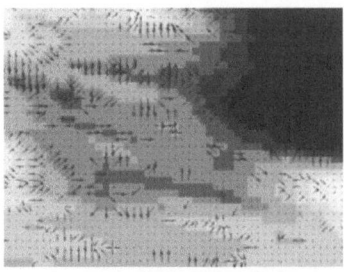

Fig. 8. Close up on figure 7.

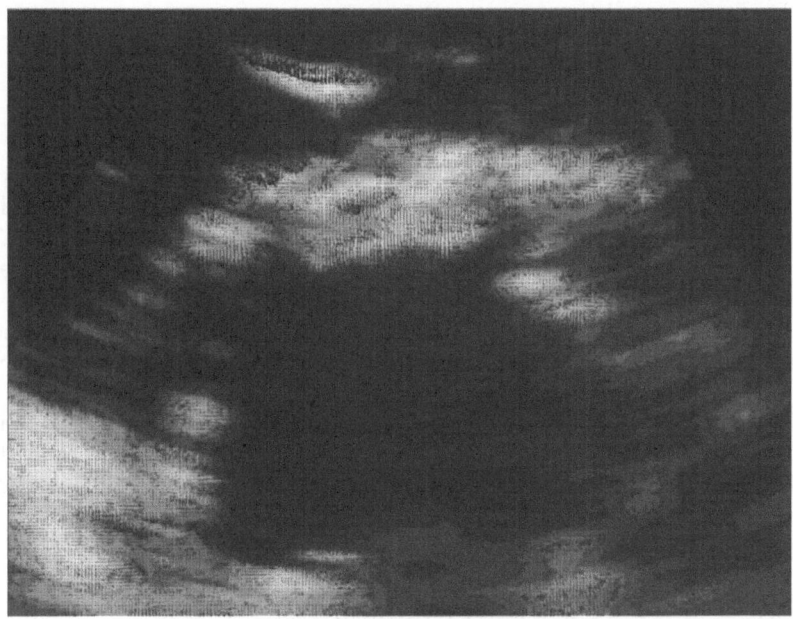

Fig. 9. Velocity field with a radiality constraint.

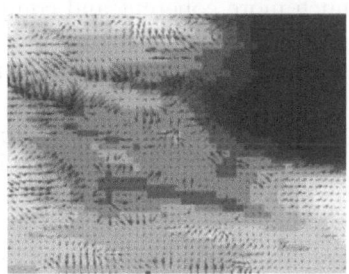

Fig. 10. Close up on figure 9.

$I_y = \frac{\partial I}{\partial y}$ and $I_t = \frac{\partial I}{\partial t}$. This is called the constraint of the optical flow. It does not define a unique solution. Our solution is inspired by the Horn and Schunck's method and will take advantage of the knowledge of the DTI information. The field we are looking for will satisfy three constraints:

1. The optical flow constraint.
2. The agreement with the DTI velocity.
3. A regularity constraint.

These properties are obtained as follows: we look for a vector field (u, v) which minimizes

$$E(u, v) = \iint_\Omega (x_{DTI}u + y_{DTI}v - v_{DTI})^2 + \alpha(\|\nabla u\|^2 + \|\nabla v\|^2)$$
$$+\beta(I_x u + I_y v + I_t)^2 dxdy$$

where α and β are positive constants, Ω is the image domain, (x_{DTI}, y_{DTI}) denotes the direction of the sensor and v_{DTI} denotes the norm of the velocity measured by the DTI. We minimize this energy with a steepest gradient descent. We used a discretization by finite differences with an explicit scheme. We give an example in the figure 5. All the examples were obtained on the same image taken during the systole. The results are satisfying compared with simple optical flow (figure 4). We get a more regular field without increasing the diffusion. We observe that the velocity field mainly represents a motion of contraction. But this field is still very noisy.

We can improve the results by using the idea of [11]. It consists of using a spatio-temporal regularization instead of a spatial regularization. It leads us to process the whole sequence simultaneously by minimizing the following energy:

$$E(u, v) = \iiint_{\Omega \times [0;T]} (x_{DTI}u + y_{DTI}v - v_{DTI})^2 + \alpha(\|\nabla u\|^2 + \|\nabla v\|^2)$$
$$+\beta(I_x u + I_y v + I_t)^2 dxdydt.$$

The rest of the algorithm is the same. An example of result is shown if figure 7. As in [11], the result is much more coherent and complete.

In order to improve results, we set soft constraints from a priori information about the heart deformation. In this type of image, the deformation is a contraction. Its center is the center of the heart. We then imposed a radiality constraint on the energy. Let $O = (x_O, y_O)$ be the center and radiuses R_1 and R_2 define a ring around the myocardium wall: $C(O, R_1, R_2) = \{(x, y), R_1 \leq d(O, (x, y)) \leq R_2\}$. We add a term to the energy of the form $\int_{[0;T]}\iint_{C(O,R_1,R_2)}(u.(x - x_o) - v.(y - y_o))^2 dxdydt$. We obtain figure 9. We can see the result of the constraint on the direction of the field but we could lose information while giving too much a priori information. The choice of adding this constraint or not is dependent on the application.

We checked the validity of our results by deforming an image with the velocity field and comparing to the following image, both visually and with a quadratic norm. This comparison gave good results, but, since we calculate a smooth field, it is not an quantitative evaluation of the quality of the velocity field. In future work, we will analyse the deformation field by the way of segmentation and classification algorithms. Then we will compare these analysis with other medical datas. That is how we will be able to check this deformation field estimation.

4   Conclusion

We have presented different ways to use the Doppler Tissue Imaging (DTI) in order to determine deformation of the cardiac wall. We first showed a way to track points along the cardiac wall in a M-Mode image (1D+t), based on a deformable grid energy minimization. We then showed how to estimate the deformation field in a sequence of 2D images (2D+t), based on energy minimization including spatio-temporal regularization and a priori constraints. Future work includes analyzing the deformation of the cardiac wall and finding pathology starting from the deformation field method we described in this paper.

References

1. L. D. Cohen, F. Pajany, D. Pellerin, and C. Veyrat. Cardiac wall tracking using doppler tissue imaging (DTI). In *In Proc. of International Conference on Image Processing (ICIP'96)*, pages III–295–298, Lausanne, Switzerland, Sept. 1996.
2. M. Bro-Nielsen. Active Nets and Cubes. *Technical Report, Institute of Mathematical Modelling, Technical University of Denmark*, Nov 1994.
3. K. Yoshino, T. Kawashima and Y. Aoki. Dynamic Reconfiguration of Active Net Structure. *Asian Conference on Computer Vision*, November 1993.
4. L.D. Cohen. On active contours models and balloons. *Computer Vision, Graphics, and Image Processing: Image Understanding*, 53(2):211-218 March 1991.
5. A. Blake, A. Zisserman, *Visual Reconstruction*. MIT Press, 1987.
6. C. Veyrat, D. Pellerin, L.D. Cohen,F. Larrazet, F. Extramiana, and S. Witchitz Spectral, one-or two-dimensional tissue velocity doppler imaging: which to choose? *Cardiology*, 9(1):9–18, 2000.
7. D. Pellerin, A. Berdeaux,L.D. Cohen,J.F. Giudicelli,S. Witchitz, and C. Veyrat, Comparison of two myocardial velocity gradient assessment methods during dobutamine infusion using doppler myocardial imaging. *Journal of the American Society of Echocardiography*, 12:22–31, 1999.
8. B.K.P. Horn and B.G. Schunck. Determining Optical Flow. *Artificial Intelligence*, (17) (1-3) :185–204, 1981.
9. G. Aubert, R. Deriche and P. Kornprobst. Optical flow estimation while preserving its dicontinuities: A variational approach. *Proceedings of the second asian conference on computer vision.*,1995
10. J.L. Barron, D.J. Fleet, S.S. Beauchemin, Performances of optical flow techniques. *International Journal of Computer Vision*, 12(1) p.43-77 (1994).
11. J. Weickert et C. Schnorr. Variational Optic Flow Computation with a Spatio-Temporal Smoothness Constraint. *Journal of Mathematical Imaging and Vision*, 14(3), May 2001.

A New Kinetic Modeling Scheme for the Human Left Ventricle Wall Motion with MR-Tagging Imaging

Cyril F. Allouche[1][*], S. Makam[1], Nicholas Ayache[2], and Hervé Delingette[2]

[1] Philips Research France, Medical Imaging Systems Group,51 rue Carnot, BP 301, 92156 Suresnes, France;
Cyril.Allouche@polytechnique.org
[2] INRIA, Projet Epidaure, 2004 Route des Lucioles, BP 93, 06902 Sophia-Antipolis, France

Abstract. Magnetic resonance tagging has proved to be an efficient non-invasive imaging technique for the study of the heart motion, producing a sharp and dense pattern on the tissues. Up to now, the quality of information derived from it has been unequalled by other modalities. It seems to be the perfect modality for the building of heart motion models. However, its main drawback was the tediousness of the image processing tasks it requires to extract the information. Recent achievements [1,9] have overcome that. In previous work [2], we have presented a novel parametric class of deformation for the 2D heart motion in the short axis planes. From it, we can compute a very accurate and compact analytical expression of the walls motion from the grid information. We present here this kinetic model, and its applications to heart modeling. In particular, we build a decomposition basis of the 2D motion with only three orthogonal modes.

1 Introduction

1.1 Tagging Protocols

Classical tagging, known as SPAMM (SPAtial Modulation of Magnetization) [14], produces a pattern (so-called *tag*), usually a grid, on the myocardial tissue, which remains along time, thus enabling to follow the motion. From Fisher's improvement CSPAMM (for Complementary SPAMM) [6], which prevents the tags from fading away, Stuber et al [13] introduced a new method which enables to track the first acquisition slice along the cycle. This is known as the "Slice Following" technique. The true in-plane 2D motion of the initial slice is hence acquired, with few artifacts. Validations of this technique to healthy and pathological hearts have already been published [12,11].

---

[*] corresponding author

T. Katila et al. (Eds.): FIMH 2001, LNCS 2230, pp. 61–68, 2001.

1.2 Motion Acquisition and Modeling

In the last decade, many works have dedicated to the acquisition of relevant kinetic parameters from tagging [3,10,7,8,4,5]. All of these methods require to use 3D geometrical models to interpolate between the acquisition slices. This induces necessarily an additive bias, as the classical SPAMM images are highly anisotropic and subject to partial volume effects. The Slice-Following technique enables to avoid these drawbacks, and permits a direct "real" 2D motion reconstruction.

In [1,2], we introduced a new algorithm which enables the fully automatic extraction of the tagging grid, in a very accurate and rapid manner. When applied to CSPAMM images, it even enables to extract the maximum intensity grid, multiplying hence the information by four. We then introduced a new parametric deformation class with which the grid motion in the short axis plane can be approximated with a very high sharpness. Moreover, the global motion parameters (rotation and contraction) are embedded in the model, and hence directly computed, for both walls. We briefly recall this deformation class, and then show an application of it: the approximation of the heart true 2D motion with only three orthogonal modes.

2 Parametric Deformation Class

2.1 Construction

The motion of the normal LV walls in the short axis planes looks very close to a similarity deformation (rotation+contraction/dilation+translation). We chose to base our model on this transformation class. To make it closer to the reality, the idea is to enable the dilation and rotation to vary smoothly along the wall. Let us consider the complex plane centered at the LV barycenter (roughly computed). We introduce the deformation which transforms a point $z = |z|e^{i\theta}$ into:

$$f_{(a_i),d}(z) = |z|\Big(\underbrace{\sum_{k=-N,k\neq0}^{N} a_k e^{ik\theta}}_{\Phi(\theta)} \Big) + d \quad , \quad (a_k) \in \mathbb{C}^{2N+1}, \quad d \in \mathbb{C} \quad (1)$$

$|a_1|$ induces the homogeneous dilation/contraction, $\arg(a_1)$ the rotation, d the translation, and all other Fourier terms stand for the "elastic perturbation". The N order is the elasticity degree of the deformation in the "Fourier sense".

2.2 Computation of the Deformation from Tagging

Let $\mathcal{C}$ be a contour (delineating a wall, the mid-myocardium, or any other line shaped zone of interest). We want to compute the deformation parameters of this contour, between times $t - 1$ and t. To do so, we weight each point of the grid decreasingly with its distance to $\mathcal{C}$ at $t-1$, and solve the Least Mean Square problem:

$$f_{(a_i),d}(z_{t-1}) = z_t \qquad (weight(z_{t-1})) \tag{2}$$

With $weight = \frac{1}{max(1,dist(z,\mathcal{C}))}$, we obtain an accurate interpolation scheme. As every point in the grid is taken into account, this scheme is also regularizing.

2.3   Radial Strain

A noteworthy property of our deformation class is that the radial strain is expressed by:

$$s_r^{\mathcal{C}}(\theta) = |\Phi^{\mathcal{C}}(\theta)| - 1 \tag{3}$$

where $\Phi^{\mathcal{C}}$ is defined in Eq. 1 for the deformation of contour $\mathcal{C}$.

2.4   Validations

We have validated our interpolation class and scheme on data acquired from 15 healthy volunteers, on a Philips Gyroscan 1.5 T [1,2]. The acquistion protocol was CSPAMM-Slice Following. The slice thickness was 8 mm, the grid spacing 4 mm, and the temporal resolution 35 ms, resulting in sequences of 16 to 20 frames for a cycle. Acquisitions were taken at basal (10 mm below the valves), apical (10 mm above the radiological apex) and equatorial (equally spaced between apex and base) planes.

We proceeded as follows: the endocardium and epicardium walls were manually segmented on the first images, then the segmentations were propagated by applying the computed deformations. Visual validations of both segmentations and particular points following were considered extremely good. The parameter curves appeared highly accurate and better than those obtained by manual techniques [11]. The average absolute error on the fitting of the grid points was 0.57 mm in radius and 1.06° in angle for the basal plane, and 0.45 mm and 1.12° for the apical plane. This does not take into account the regularization effect of the deformation, over the error embedded in the grid.

$N = 3$ appeared as the optimal order of the deformation, providing both sufficient elasticity and regularization. $N > 3$ is indeed "too elastic" for the noise level of the grid information, while $N < 3$ underfits the motion.

2.5   Acquisition of Clinical and Kinematic Parameters

As we dispose of an explicit analytical expression of the deformation at each phase, we can compute any parameter of clinical or modeling relevance (lumen surface, shortening profile, local motion amplitude, etc ... [12,11]). Moreover, the a_1 coefficient carries a huge kinetic sense: it provides, by construction, the best similarity approximation of the motion. Curves of temporal evolution of its modulus and argument are of great interest for both clinical and modeling purposes. See figures 1 and 2 for an example.

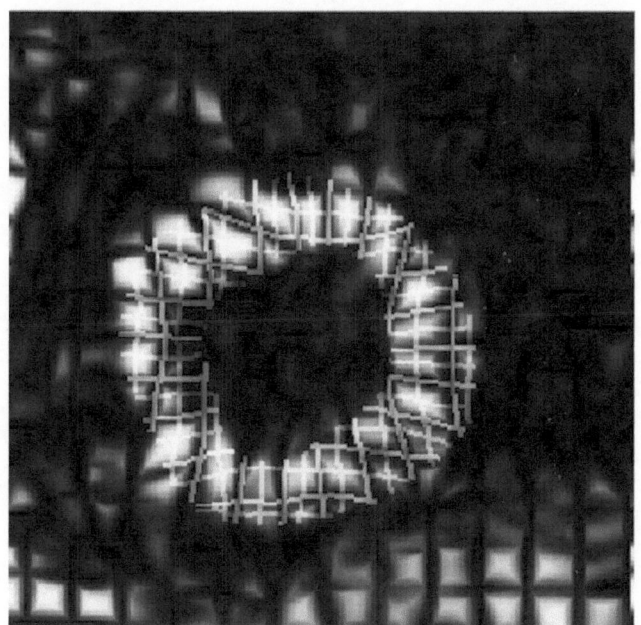

Fig. 1. Example of Tag Extraction Used for Validations (Basal)

3   Towards a Compact Kinetic Model

3.1   Complex Principal Component Analysis

With $N = 3$, our deformation is guided by 7 complex parameters, which is rather compact related to the high degree of accuracy it handles. However, the main component of the motion is mainly controlled by the similarity coefficients a_1 and d, the rest being an elastic complement. We propose to reduce *a posteriori* this 5-parameter term to a single mode of variation on a cycle, for a same patient and same slice. Let C_t be the $(a_k)_{k=-3\ldots3}$ vector at time t. Let us consider the classical hermitian product: $< A|B > = \overline{A^t}B$. If $t = 0$ is the reference time, $C_0 = (0\ldots a_1 = 1\quad 0\ldots0)$. Then $< C_0|C_t > C_0 = (0\ldots a_1^t\quad 0\ldots0)$ stands for the projection of C_t on the subspace of the similarities . Let now consider

$$B_t = \frac{C_t - < C_0|C_t > C_0}{< C_0|C_t >} \tag{4}$$

B_t stands hence for the non-semi-rigid part of the deformation C_t, semi-rigidly registered to C_0.

A Principal Component Analysis (in $\mathbb{C}$) of $(B_t)_{t=0..t_n}$ leads to:

$$B_t \simeq M_0 + < V_0|B_t > V_0 \tag{5}$$

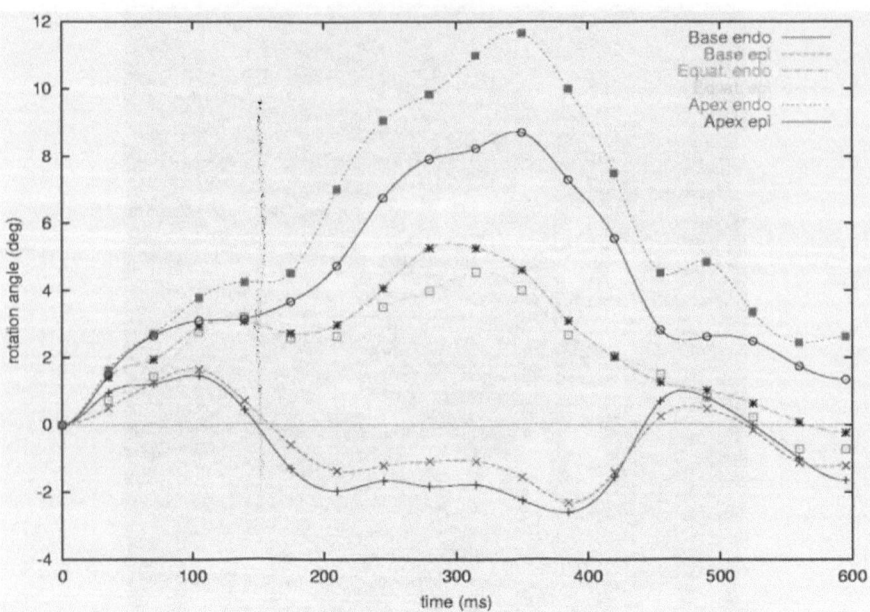

Fig. 2. Twist Computation for the Endo- and Epi-cardial Walls, at the Basal, Equatorial and Apical Levels

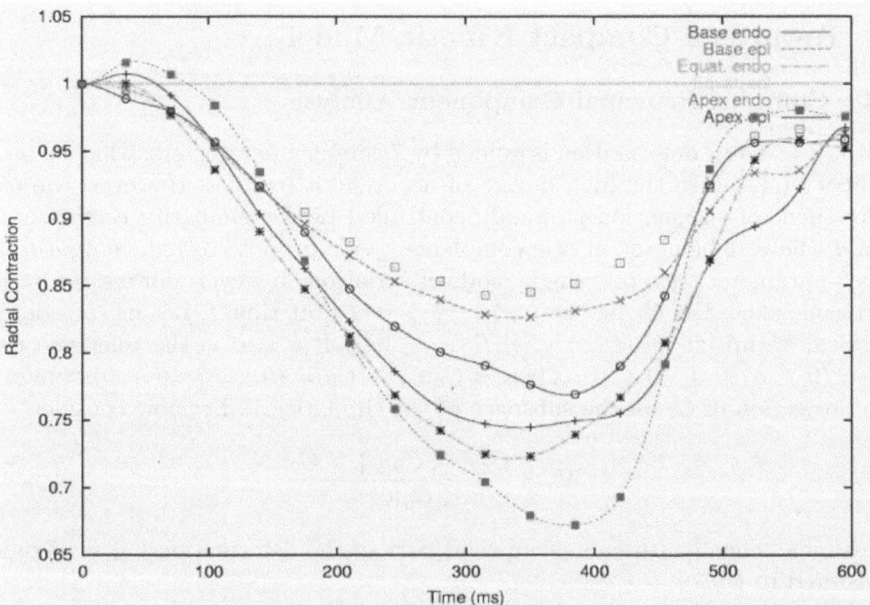

Fig. 3. Computation of Radial Contraction for the Endo- and Epi-cardial Walls, at the Basal, Equatorial and Apical Levels

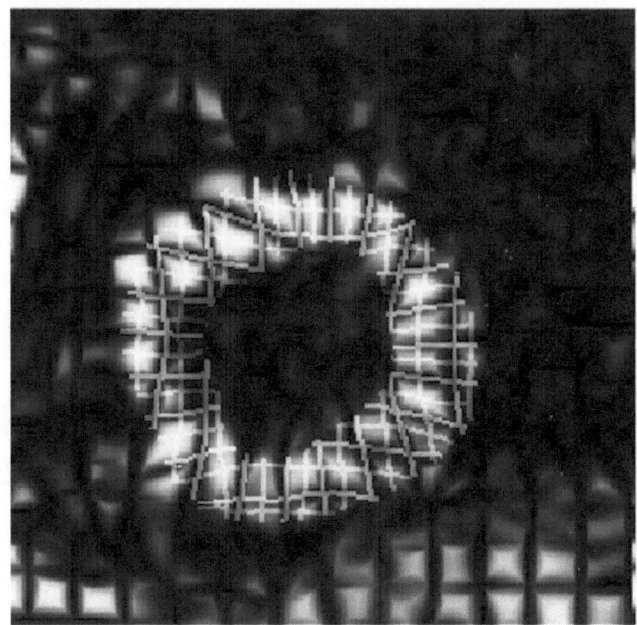

Fig. 1. Example of Tag Extraction Used for Validations (Basal)

3   Towards a Compact Kinetic Model

3.1   Complex Principal Component Analysis

With $N = 3$, our deformation is guided by 7 complex parameters, which is rather compact related to the high degree of accuracy it handles. However, the main component of the motion is mainly controlled by the similarity coefficients a_1 and d, the rest being an elastic complement. We propose to reduce *a posteriori* this 5-parameter term to a single mode of variation on a cycle, for a same patient and same slice. Let C_t be the $(a_k)_{k=-3\ldots3}$ vector at time t. Let us consider the classical hermitian product: $< A|B > = \overline{A^t}B$. If $t = 0$ is the reference time, $C_0 = (0 \ldots a_1 = 1 \quad 0 \ldots 0)$. Then $< C_0|C_t > C_0 = (0 \ldots a_1^t \quad 0 \ldots 0)$ stands for the projection of C_t on the subspace of the similarities . Let now consider

$$B_t = \frac{C_t - < C_0|C_t > C_0}{< C_0|C_t >} \tag{4}$$

B_t stands hence for the non-semi-rigid part of the deformation C_t, semi-rigidly registered to C_0.

A Principal Component Analysis (in $\mathbb{C}$) of $(B_t)_{t=0..t_n}$ leads to:

$$B_t \simeq M_0 + < V_0|B_t > V_0 \tag{5}$$

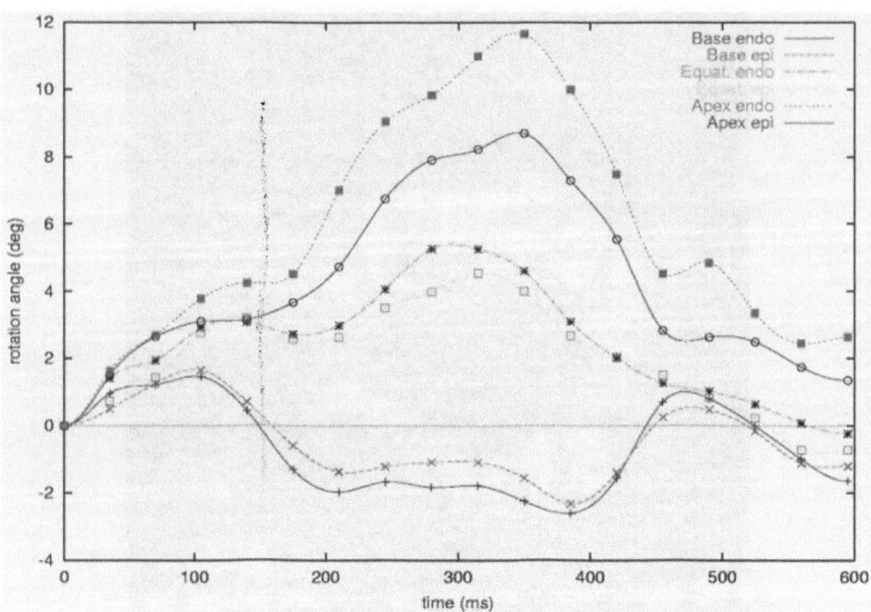

Fig. 2. Twist Computation for the Endo- and Epi-cardial Walls, at the Basal, Equatorial and Apical Levels

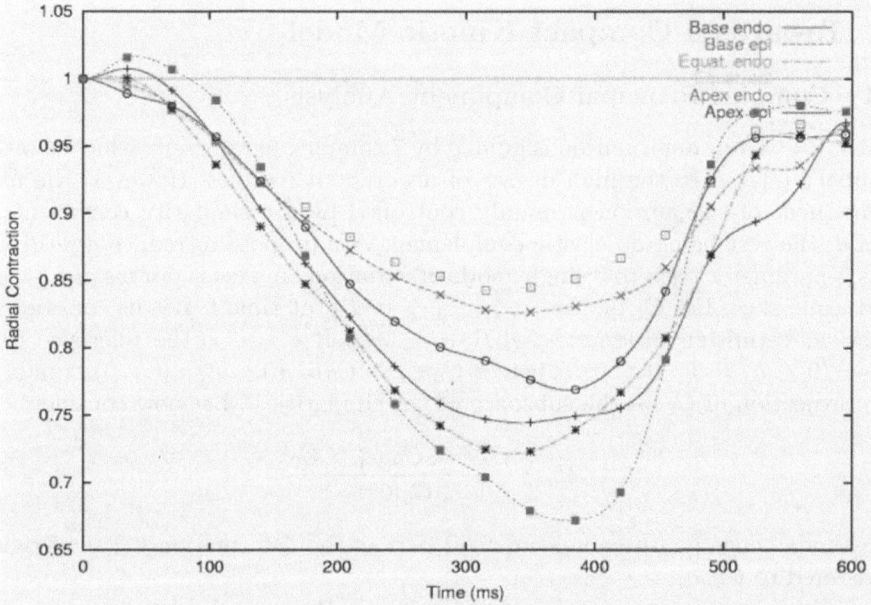

Fig. 3. Computation of Radial Contraction for the Endo- and Epi-cardial Walls, at the Basal, Equatorial and Apical Levels

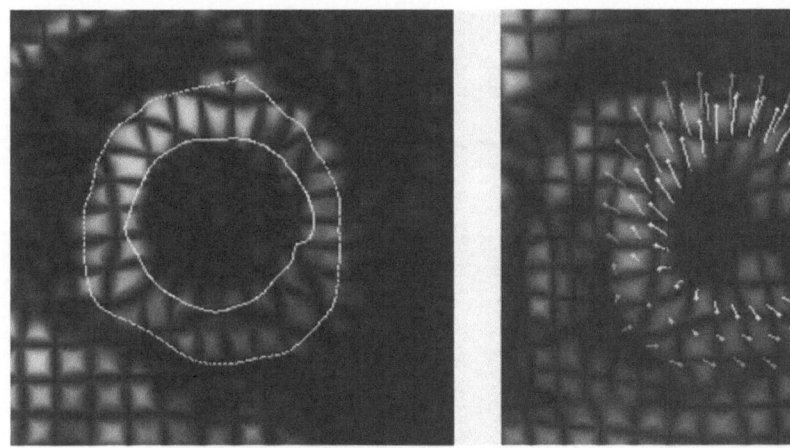

Fig. 4. Left: Propagation of Segmentation (Basal, End-Systole). Right: Motion from Early to End-Diastole, at Basal Level, for Endocardium, Epicardium and Mid-Myocardium

where M_0 is the mean vector of B_t, and V_0 the normalized first eigenvector. Calculations on our datasets of healthy patients proved that the mean vector M_0 is always negligible, and that the first eigenvector has a very high weight related to the other ones.

As, by construction, B_t is orthogonal to C_0, so is V_0, and then we can rewrite, returning to vector C_t:

$$C_t \simeq < C_0 | C_t > C_0 + < V_0 | C_t > V_0 \tag{6}$$

Finally, by returning to Eq. 1, we obtain:

$$f_{(a_i),d}(z) \simeq g_{a_1,d,\lambda}(z) = \underbrace{\boldsymbol{a_1}z + \boldsymbol{d}}_{Similarity} + \underbrace{\boldsymbol{\lambda}|z| \sum_{k=-3,k\neq 0}^{3} v_0^k e^{ik\theta}}_{Elastic} \quad , \quad \theta = \arg(z) \tag{7}$$

We then have an *a posteriori* orthogonal decomposition of the motion with three parameters: $a_1(t), d(t), \lambda(t)$.

3.2   Physiological Interpretation

After preliminary results on our volunteers database, we have observed that the V_0 eigenvector representing the elastic deformation had always similar shapes, its temporal influence being a unimodal curve, with maximum around the end-systole, and its spatial influence being maximal on three anatomical points: the two junctions of the right ventricle (RV), and the middle of the lateral wall. See Fig. 5. Physiologically, this can be interpreted by the fact that the septal

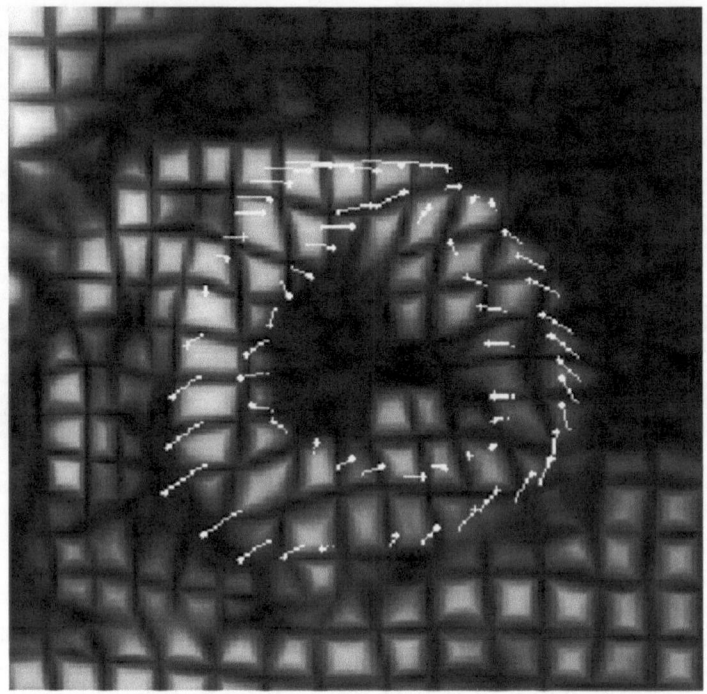

Fig. 5. Elastic Part of the Motion, for Both Walls, at End-Systole, Basal Shot. Scale *4 for Visibility

wall has a diphasic motion, taking part in both the LV and the RV motions, while the lateral wall is almost free of influence from the RV. In a sense, the RV perturbates the LV motion from a perfect similarity.

4   Conclusion

We have presented a new parametric deformation class from which the 2D motion of the Left Ventricle in the short axis planes can be very sharply approximated and modeled. Coupled with the "CSPAMM-Slice Following" tagging technique, it enables to compute the true motion of the left ventricle in the short axis plane.

By analyzing our deformation parameters, we have showed that the non-rigid part of the motion can be reduced to a single-mode deformation, which can be physiologically interpreted.

The three-orthogonal-mode decomposition of the motion we obtain will be of great help in many image processing tasks, including 2D registration and motion computation in non-marked images, as also in model-guided segmentation.

Our method was very recently extended to 4D modeling, and very promising results have already been obtained.

Acknowledgments. The authors wish to thank the Beth Israel Deaconess Medical Center, Boston (MA) and the Institute of Biomedical Engineering and Medical Informatics of the Zurich University and ETH, Zurich (Switzerland) for the medical data, and Philips Medical Systems, Best (the Netherlands), for technical support.

References

1. CF Allouche. Automatic, Real-time Processing of SPAMM-tagged Myocardium Images. In *8th Annual Conference of the International Society for Magnetic Resonance in Medicine*, page 830. ISMRM, April 2001. ISSN 1524-6965.
2. CF Allouche, S Makram-Ebeid, M Stuber, N Ayache, and H Delingette. New Methods and Algorithms for the Accurate, Real-time, Motion Analysis of the Left Ventricle with MRI-Tagging. In *Proc. Computer Assisted Radiology and Surgery (CARS)*, volume 1230 of *Excerpta Medica International Congress Series*, pages 911–916. Elsevier, June 2001.
3. AA Amini, RW Curwen, and JC Gore. Snakes and splines for tracking nonrigid heart motion. In *Proc.Eur.Conf.Computer Vision*, pages 251–261, Cambridge,UK, Apr. 1996.
4. P Clarysse, D Friboulet, and IE Magnin. Tracking geometrical descriptors on 3D deformable surfaces: Application to the left ventricular surface of the heart. *IEEE Trans.Med.Imag.*, 16(4):392–404, 1997.
5. J Declerck, J Feldmar, and N Ayache. Definition of a 4D continuous planispheric transformation for the tracking and the analysis of LV motion. *Medical Image Analysis*, 2(2):197–213, 1998.
6. SE Fischer, GC McKinnon, SE Maier, and P Boesiger. Improved Myocardial Tagging Contrast. *Magn Reson Med*, 30:191–200, 1993.
7. D Friboulet, IE Magnin, and D Revel. Assessment of a model for overall left ventricular three-dimensional motion from MRI data. *Intl.Journal of Cardiac Imaging*, 8:175–90, 1992.
8. T McInerney and D Terzopoulos. A finite element model for 3D shape reconstruction and nonrigid motion tracking. In *Proc. 4th International Conference on Computer Vision*, pages 518–23, 1993.
9. N Osman, W Kerwin, E McVeigh, and J Prince. Cardiac motion tracking using CINE harmonic phase HARP magnetic resonance imaging. *Magn.Res. in Medicine*, 42:1048–1060, 1999.
10. J Park, D Metaxas, AA Young, and L Axel. Analysis of Left Ventricular Wall Motion Based on Volumetric Deformable Models and MRI-SPAMM. *Medical Image Analysis*, 1(1), 1996.
11. M Stuber, E Nagel, SE Fisher, MA Spiegel, MB Scheidegger, and P Boesiger. Quantification of the local heartwall motion by magnetic resonance myocardial tagging. *Comp. Med. Imag. Graph.*, 22:217–228, 1998.
12. M Stuber, MB Scheidegger, and SE Fischer. Alterations in the local myocardial motion pattern in patients suffering from pressure overload due to aortic stenosis. *Circulation*, 100:361–8, 1999.
13. M Stuber, MA Spiegel, and SE Fischer. Single breath-hold slice-following CSPAMM myocardial tagging. *Magma*, 9:85–91, 1999.
14. EA Zerhouni, DM Parish, WJ Rogers, A Yang, and EP Shapiro. Human heart: tagging with MR imaging- a method for noninvasive assessment of myocardial motion. *Radiology*, (169):56–59, 1988.

Integrated Quantitative Analysis of Tagged Magnetic Resonance Images

Patrick Clarysse, Pierre Croisille, Luc Bracoud, and Isabelle Magnin

CREATIS, UMR CNRS #5515,
F-69621 Villeurbanne, France
{patrick.clarysse, pierre.croisille, luc.bracoud,
isabelle.magnin}@creatis.insa-lyon.fr

Abstract. An image processing pipeline is presented for the quantitative analysis of 2D grid tagged Magnetic Resonance images. The first step concerns the automatic extraction of the tagging pattern and the definition of the left ventricular myocardial contours. In a second step, a spatio-temporal displacement field is fitted to the tag data points. Finally, parameters related to the contractile function can be investigated through graphic displays, movies and statistical analysis.

1 Introduction

Magnetic Resonance (MR) tagging is a technique of choice for analyzing the motion of the heart. Since the introduction of the technique more than ten years ago [1], a great number of methods have been published for the processing of 2D and 3D tagged images [2-10]. Up to now, despite the availability of MR tagging sequences on most MR scanners, no standard tool has been commonly adopted for the quantitative analysis of the heart motion from MR tagging. In fact, the quantitative analysis of tagged MR Images requires several successive steps (Figure 1) each of which having to be carefully validated. In a previous work, we have proposed a simple approach for fitting a spatio-temporal displacement field [10] from which several parameters related to the mechanics of the myocardium can be derived. Some tools have also been developed for the analysis of parameter sets in order to detect contraction abnormalities [12].

In this paper, we describe the processing scheme, named *TagAnalyze,* for the complete analysis of 2D + time tagged data from the acquisition to the computer aided diagnosis of contractile abnormalities.

2 Processing Pipeline of Tagged MR Images

TagAnalyze is a processing pipeline for 2D tagged MR Image sequences. It handles grid tagged images in order to extract clinically relevant parameters. Figure 1 illustrates the main steps of the processing pipeline, which are detailed in the subsequent

T. Katila et al. (Eds.): FIMH 2001, LNCS 2230, pp. 69-75, 2001.
© Springer-Verlag Berlin Heidelberg 2001

subsections. Three examinations were considered in this study : one healthy volunteer, two ischemic patients at rest and under pharmacological stress.

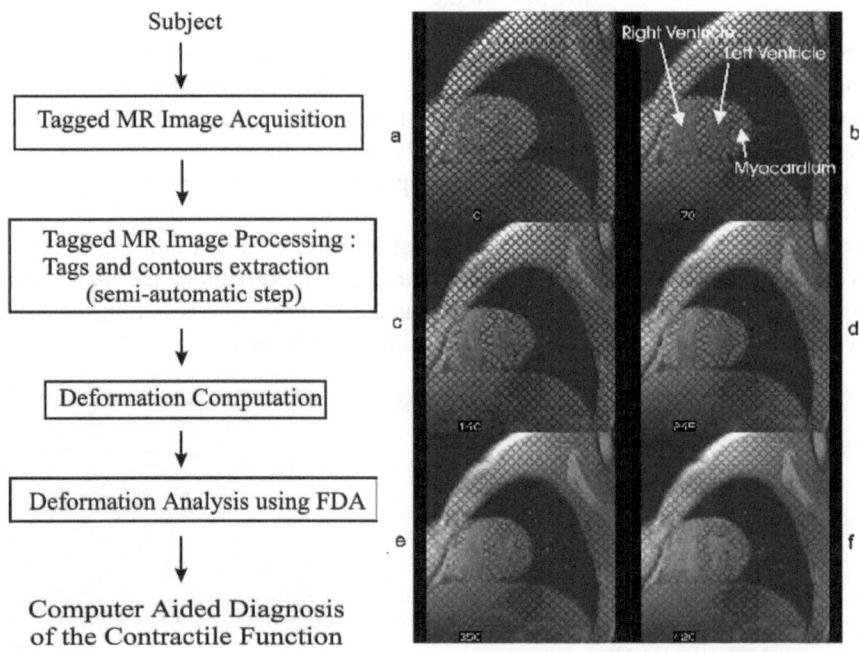

Fig. 1. Main steps of the processing pipeline of the tagged MR images from acquisition to diagnosis. A short axis slice at six instants through the cardiac systole (a-f) is shown on the right. FDA stands for "functional data analysis".

2.1 Tags and Contours Extraction

Our approach requires the extraction of the tagging pattern and of the left ventricular (LV) contours. First, a Region of Interest (ROI) is interactively defined. A cine loop of the image sequence allows the user to check the appropriateness of the ROI location and size. Then, a myocardial mask is defined by the manual tracing of the epicardial contour onto the end-diastolic image and of the endocardial contour onto the end-systolic image. Extraction of the tags and displacement calculation will be performed within the region given by the mask.

Extraction of the tagging pattern is based on the concept of active meshes [13-15]. The initial position of the grid tagging pattern is interactively defined. Each tag direction is defined one after the other by tracing a line onto the image. Intersections (nodes) of the grid are automatically derived and a mesh structure is sent to the tag extraction algorithm (Figure 2). Each node is assimilated to a particle of mass m linked to its neighbors with springs (stiffness k). The spring net, initially at rest, is submitted to an external force field originating from the tagged image. An equilibrium is reached when the following global energy is minimized :

$$M\ddot{U} + C\dot{U} + KU = F(t)$$

where M is the mass matrix, C the damping diagonal matrix (damping force is proportional to the velocity and defined by the constant c), K is the stiffness matrix (the stiffness of the springs is set to k), F is the force matrix and U the matrix of the node displacements. The set of linear equations is solved using finite differences and an iterative process. The external force field is computed from the image itself by a Canny-Deriche gradient operator. Note that nodes outside the myocardial mask are fixed by setting their mass to infinity while nodes that are inside have a unit mass. Also, the convergence process is interruptible so that interactive corrections are made possible (automatic process can be resumed after manual editing). The resulting mesh at the current frame is used as the initial solution for the next frame.

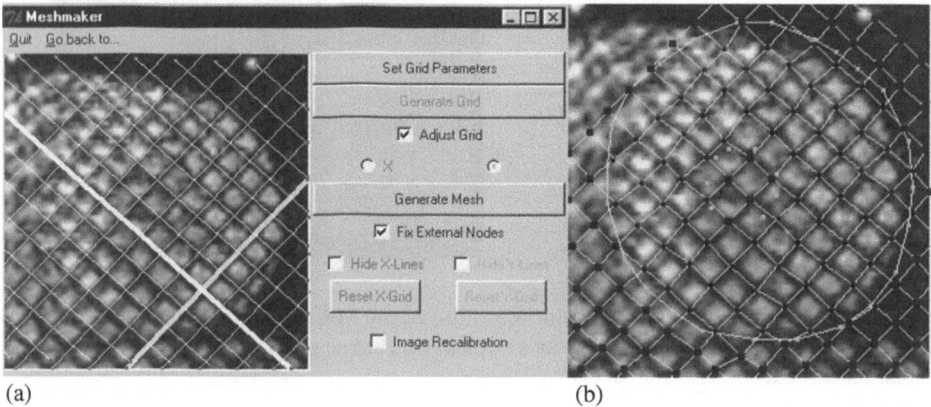

(a)   (b)

Fig. 2. (a) Definition of the initial regular mesh. (b) Resulting mesh at convergence on the first frame (end-diastole) for the healthy subject.

The tags' location is further refined using an active contour which is a simple and fast geometrical model similar to the discrete dynamic contour model of Lobregt and Viergever [16]. It is applied individually on each tag line which is first subdivided and constrained in the vicinity of the original segments (Figure 3). Usually, 30 iterations are sufficient and the process rapidly ends up when the speed of the contour points is close to zero. This step is important because each tag line is defined by a limited number of points within the active mesh. The smoothing step adds points to the tag lines and regularizes their shape while constraining them to lie inside the tag valleys. The consistency through space and time of the tags is verified with a cine-loop. At any stage, user interaction is allowed. The tag points within the myocardial mask for each frame are finally saved in a file.

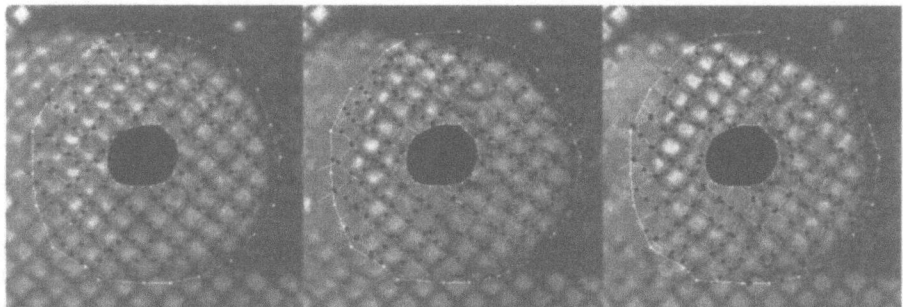

Fig. 3. Smoothed tag lines using the discrete dynamic contour model in the first three frames of the healthy subject.

2.2   Displacement Field Estimation

A spatio-temporal displacement field is fitted to the tag points using the algorithm described in [10]. Briefly, the components of the inverse displacement field (from deformed state to the reference undeformed state) are first estimated by computing the parameters of a hierarchical cosine series model. Using the correspondences given by this model, the parameters of the direct displacement field are calculated. Optimal model orders have been derived from an accuracy study as a function of the tagging pattern parameters [10].

One advantage of such a parametric model is that it allows for the straightforward calculation of motion related parameters such as deformation tensors, principal deformations, speed and acceleration. The mean global translation is subtracted in order to keep only the deformation part of the myocardial media. Displacement and deformation tensors are displayed using the *fur-like* representation based on 2D texture synthesis [17] where the fibers encode the orientation, direction, and magnitude (color) of the vectors (Figure 4).

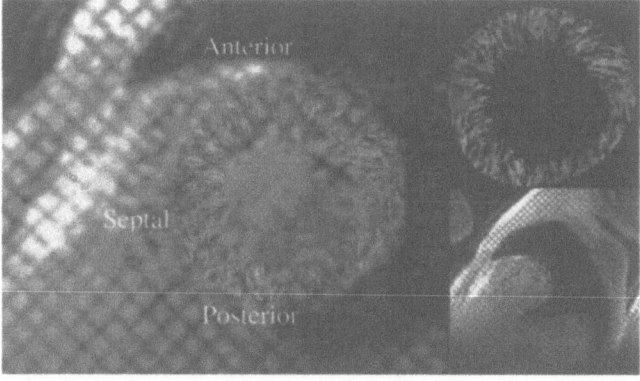

Fig. 4. Representation of the displacement field at end-systole for patient P2 at rest with the fur-like representation (spatial orders = 5, temporal order = 7).

The concatenation of the representation at each time point of the cardiac cycle allows for the visualization of the temporal evolution of the parameters.

2.3   Analysis of the Contractile Function

The previous step provides a wealth of information that needs to be summed up for the clinician. Evolution of deformation parameters can be displayed using multi-box plots and bull's eye representations. Figure 5 shows the temporal evolution of the maximum shortening at midwall and for the medium level with the healthy subject and the pathological case P1. Statistical tools have been developed in order to ease the analysis of the parameters through examinations. In particular, a healthy subject database has been studied to derive a statistical model of the normal contraction pattern from which a given patient can be compared to. Interested readers are referred to [11-12].

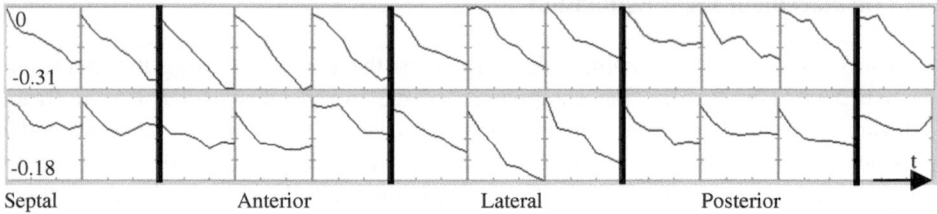

Septal   Anterior   Lateral   Posterior

Fig. 5. Evolution of the Maximum Shortening at a medium level for the healthy subject (up) and patient P1 at rest (bottom).

3   Implementation Considerations

The programs related to the tagged image processing and the displacement field fitting have been written in C-C++ language and embedded in a Tcl-Tk[1] user interface. Some graphical functions make use of the Vtk[2] library. It is therefore platform independent and do not require any commercial libraries.

The automatic steps (active mesh and contours) of the tags and contours extraction from one 2D tagged sequence are very fast (a few seconds). User control is still required especially at the mask borders. Less than 3 minutes are needed for the spatio-temporal model estimation with the optimal orders (Spatial orders = 5, temporal order = 7, 9 phases) including the generation of the displacement field representations on a Pentium III, 800MHz.

---

[1] Ajuba Solutions
[2] Visualization ToolKit.

4 Discussion and Conclusion

We have presented the 2D tagged image processing pipeline, *TagAnalyze*. Two dimensional grid tagged images can be fully exploited within a reasonable amount of time. The extraction of the tagging pattern is fast but still requires user control. We have insisted on the importance of the tag smoothing step. Its impact onto the displacement field fitting could be evaluated. Note that multi-slice short axis acquisitions, covering the LV, can be treated by the pipeline as well.

The remaining important problem of this pipeline concerns the automatic extraction of the endocardial and epicardial contours which was manually performed by the definition of a mask. The mask edges need not be accurate for the displacement field computation. In practice, we usually overestimate the LV epicardial border while underestimating the endocardial border. Although not crucial for the calculation of the myocardial deformation, accurate definition of the LV contours is required for the interpretation of the results. The automatic LV segmentation is a non trivial task since the tags blur the contours. If no standard cine acquisition is available, one needs to preprocess the images in order to clear up the tags. Denney overcomes the problem of myocardial contour identification introducing the ML/MAP method for the identification of tags without user defined contours [8]. It is based on the physics of the tagging process and on signal intensity and noise statistics computed from image data. The method has been applied to parallel tag patterns. In our method, only a crude estimate of the inner and outer LV contours is used to define a ROI. The MAP hypothesis test introduced in [8] could be used to improve a posteriori the definition of the contours at each phase.

An original heart motion estimation method that uses harmonic phase (HARP) images as been proposed by Osman et al. [9]. This method relies on basic mathematical operations and is therefore fast. It allows for the reconstruction of displacement fields for small motions. Comparison of both approaches would be particularly interesting.

The extension of the pipeline to process 3D tagged images implies the adaptation of the pipeline for the treatment of long axis images. The checking of the consistency of the 3D tags in space and time would necessitate 3D visualization tools. Based on the same principle, the extension of the displacement field computation algorithm has been performed but, since the process has not yet been optimized, the 3D computation is time consuming.

TagAnalyze is currently involved in the study of patients suffering of hypertrophic myocardial diseases.

Acknowledgments. This work was performed within the framework of the joint incentive action "Beating Heart" of the research groups ISIS, ALP and MSPC of the French National Center for Scientific Research (CNRS). It is partly granted by the Région Rhône Alpes, through the AdéMO project and by the Lipha Santé Company, a subsidiary of the group MERCK KGaA. The authors are grateful to Meimei Han and Christophe Basset for their contribution to this work.

References

[1]   E. A. Zerhouni, D. M. Parish, W. J. Rogers, A. Yang, and E. P. Shapiro, "Human heart: tagging with MR imaging - A method for noninvasive assessment of myocardial motion," *Radiology*, vol. 169, pp. 59-63, 1988.

[2]   C. C. Moore, "Calculation of three-dimensional left ventricular strains from biplanar tagged MR images," *Journal of Magnetic Resonance Imaging*, vol. March/April, pp. 165-175, 1992.

[3]   W. G. O'Dell, C. C. Moore, W. C. Hunter, E. A. Zerhouni, and E. R. McVeigh, "Three-dimensional myocardial deformations: calculation with displacement field fitting to tagged MR images," *Radiology*, vol. 195, pp. 829-835, 1995.

[4]   M. A. Guttman, J. L. Prince, and E. R. McVeigh , "Tag and contour detection in tagged MR images of the left ventricle," *IEEE Transactions on Medical Imaging*, vol. 13, N°1, pp. 74-88, 1994.

[5]   D. L. Kraitchman, A. A. Young, C.-N. Chang, and L. Axel, "Semi-automatic tracking of myocardial motion in MR tagged images," IEEE Trans. Medical Imaging, vol. 14, N° 3, pp. 422-433, 1995.

[6]   J. Park, D. Metaxas, A. A. Young, and L. Axel, "Deformable models with parameter functions for cardiac motion analysis from tagged MRI data," *IEEE Transactions on Medical Imaging*, vol. 15, N° 1, pp. 178-289, 1996.

[7]   J. Declerck, N. Ayache, and E. R. Mc Veigh, "Use of a 4D planispheric transformation for the tracking and the analysis of LV motion with tagged MR images," INRIA Tech. Rep. RR-3535, October 1998.

[8]   T. S. Denney, "Estimation and detection of myocardial tags in MR image without user-defined myocardial contours," *IEEE Transactions on Medical Imaging*, vol. 18, N° 4, pp. 330-344, 1999.

[9]   N. F. Osman, E. R. Mc Veigh, and J. L. Prince, "Imaging heart motion using harmonic phase MRI," *IEEE Transactions on Medical Imaging*, vol. 19, N° 3, pp. 186-202, 2000.

[10] P. Clarysse, C. Basset, L. Khouas, P. Croisille, D. Friboulet, C. Odet, and I. E. Magnin, "2D Spatial and temporal displacement and deformation field fitting from cardiac MR tagging," *MEDIA*, vol. 3, pp. 253-268, 2000.

[11] P. Clarysse, M. Han, P. Croisille, and I. E. Magnin, "Exploratory analysis of the spatio-temporal deformation of the myocardium during systole from tagged MRI," Biomedical Engineering Society Annual Meeting, Seattle, Washington, USA, 2000.

[12] M. Han, "Analyse exploratoire de la déformation spatio-temporelle du myocarde à partir de l'imagerie par résonance magnétique de marquage tissulaire," PhD Thesis, *INSA*. Lyon, 1999, 201p.

[13] M. Vasilescu and D. Terzopoulos, "Adaptive meshes and shells," Computer Vision and Pattern Recognition, Urbana Champain, Illinnois, USA, 1992.

[14] Y. Wang and O. Lee, "Active mesh - A feature seeking and tracking image sequence representation scheme," *IEEE Transactions on Image Processing*, vol. 3, N° 5, pp. 610-624, 1994.

[15] C. Nastar and N. Ayache, "Frequency-based nonrigid motion analysis : application to four dimensional medical images," *IEEE Transactions on Pattern Analysis and Machine Intelligence*, vol. 18, N° 1, pp. 1067-1079, 1996.

[16] S. Lobregt and M. A. Viergever, "A discrete dynamic contour model," *IEEE Transactions on Medical Imaging*, vol. 14, N° 1, pp. 12-24, 1995.

[17] L. Khouas, P. Clarysse, D. Friboulet, and C. Odet, "Fast 2D vector field visualization using a 2D texture synthesis based on an autoregressive filter. Application to cardiac imaging," *Machine Graphics and Vision*, vol. 7, N° 4, pp. 751-764, 1998.

Measurement of Ventricular Wall Motion, Epicardial Electrical Mapping, and Myocardial Fiber Angles in the Same Heart

Elliot McVeigh*, Owen Faris, Dan Ennis, Patrick Helm, and Frank Evans

Laboratory of Cardiac Energetics
National Heart Lung and Blood Institute
National Institutes of Health
Bethesda, MD
and
Johns Hopkins University School of Medicine

Abstract. Methods for the precise measurement of three dimensional myocardial motion non-invasivley with MRI have recently been developed. These methods use a technique called "presaturation tagging" to mark the myocardium, and rapid MRI to track the motion of these markers. A unique capability of this method is the production of strain images representing the local deformation of the myocardium. These images clearly show the sequence of events during the activation of the heart, and can demonstrate abnormalities caused by asynchronous electrical activation or ischemia. Coupled with the near simultaneous mapping of electrical depolarization with an epicardial sock array, we can investigate the relationship between electical activity and mechanical function on a local level. Registered fiber angle maps can be obtained in the same heart with diffusion MRI to assist in the construction of the mechano-electrical model of the whole heart.

1 Introduction

The ability to measure the precise mechanical function, the electrical function, and the underlying fiber architecture in the same heart in vivo may uncover the interactions of these constituents in normal and abnormal cardiac function.

The measurement of the electrical activity of the heart is a mature field of research employing intra-cavity electrodes [8], baskets, optical techniques [13], monophasic action potentials [5] and body surface electrode mapping [2,3,9] among other techniques.

---

* Correspondence: Elliot R. McVeigh, PhD. NHLBI, Building 10, Room B1D416, Bethesda, MD, 20892
phone: 301-496-1184, fax: 801-912-3292, email: emcveigh@bme.jhu.edu

T. Katila et al. (Eds.): FIMH 2001, LNCS 2230, pp. 76-82, 2001.
© Springer-Verlag Berlin Heidelberg 2001

Methods for measuring local three dimensional myocardial motion non-invasively with MRI have been developed using presaturation tagging patterns [1,10,17]. Recently, methods for measuring the diffusion tensor in vivo have lead to a method for measuring the fiber angle in soft tissue [6,14].

An experimental protocol has recently been developed in which electrical mapping, myocardial strain mapping and fiber angle mapping can be achieved in the same heart [4]. The data are registered so that local correlations can be made between these three features.

2 Cardiac Tagging Techniques

In cardiac tagging a set of saturation pulses placed in the tissue provides a signal intensity pattern in the tissue; the change in shape of the intensity pattern in the image reflects the change in shape of the underlying body containing the intensity pattern. Originally demonstrated by Zerhouni et. al. [17] with saturation pulses, and by Axel with SPAMM pulses [1], it was shown that parallel lines can be used to mark the tissue effectively.

The objective of the analysis of tagged images is to track the 3D motion of each material point in the heart, and then to compute the six components of the strain tensor at each point for a sequence of time points throughout the heart cycle. The strain tensor characterizes the local deformation of the myocardium. Bulk translations and rotations of the entire heart may actually dominate the displacement and velocity measurements, but these are of limited value as an index of local myocardial contraction. In order to obtain precise quantification of the regional strains, the position of the tags must be measured with a "tag detection" algorithm [7]. Once the relative position of the tags have been determined as a function of time, these data can be used to estimate the strain tensor at each point in the myocardium. One method for doing this is a displacement field model based on B-splines [12].

3 Measurement of Myocardial Function During Asynchronous Activation

In order to evaluate the relationship between electrical excitation and the onset of mechanical contraction, MR tagging experiments were performed during ectopic pacing in anesthetized normal dogs [4,11,15]. When systolic contraction was evoked by right atrial pacing, the LV was excited via the normal pathway of the Purkinje system and the pattern of mechanical activation was found to be very uniform as a function of position. However, when the heart was paced from a ventricular site, significant asynchronous and spatially heterogeneous contraction was observed.

The precise sequence of events during ectopic excitation was particularly evident on the strain images. Fig. 1 shows the evolution in time of the circumferential component of the 3D strain tensor (Ecc) evaluated at the mid-wall for two pacing sites; because the fiber direction is essentially circumferential at the midwall, this component of the strain tensor closely matches muscle fiber shortening. During atrial pacing the ventricle is activated through the normal Purkinje pathway and muscle shortening evolves relatively homogeneously over the ventricle; this is demonstrated with the uniformly increasing blue color over the ventricle in the top row of Fig. 1. With epicardial ventricular pacing, early mechanical activation was observed at the pacing site, followed by propagation of a contraction wave-front to the opposite side of the heart. This is seen as the blue "wave" of muscle shortening emanating from the RV freewall pacing site in the second row of Fig. 1. There was also a significant "prestretch" of the late activated myocardium on the opposite side of the heart from the pacing site, shown as a bright yellow color. This prestretch was quite pronounced (15–20% in some cases) and occurred in the first 100ms after the ventricular pacing pulse.

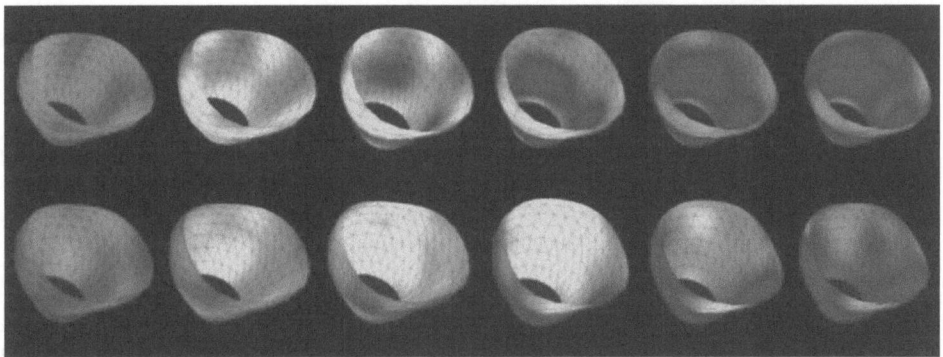

Fig. 1. These colorized surfaces show the circumferential stretch and contraction of the midwall of the myocardium; the RV extends from 5 o'clock to 10 o'clock. This surface runs through the LV and RV. The top row shows the initial stretch during filling (yellow color) and a uniform contraction over the entire heart (blue color). The bottom row shows the same heart during ectopic pacing on the epicardial surface of the RV. The LV freewall udergoes a stretch during RV contraction, contracting after a delay of approximately 100ms.

An alternative way of visualizing the contraction pattern is to graph the time course of strain for each material point of the LV. Each graph can be mapped to a position in an array that corresponds to a position in the LV. An example of such a *LV strain map* is shown in Fig. 2 where the sequence of circumferential stretching and shortening (mid-wall Ecc) for selected midwall sites in the LV freewall and the RV freewall. The points shown ar subsampled from a larger array of data. The LV strain evolution maps are an excellent method for observing the delay to the onset of contraction for different regions of the heart.

While asynchronous mechanical activation is obvious from both the color encoded strain images shown in Fig. 1 and the LV strain map showing Ecc vs. time in Fig. 2, we can also define the "mechanical activation time" as the time at which the muscle begins to shorten. This will correspond to the time at which the prestretch or ventricular filling reaches a peak and myocardial shortening begins, as shown by the red vertical lines in the LV strain maps of Fig. 2.

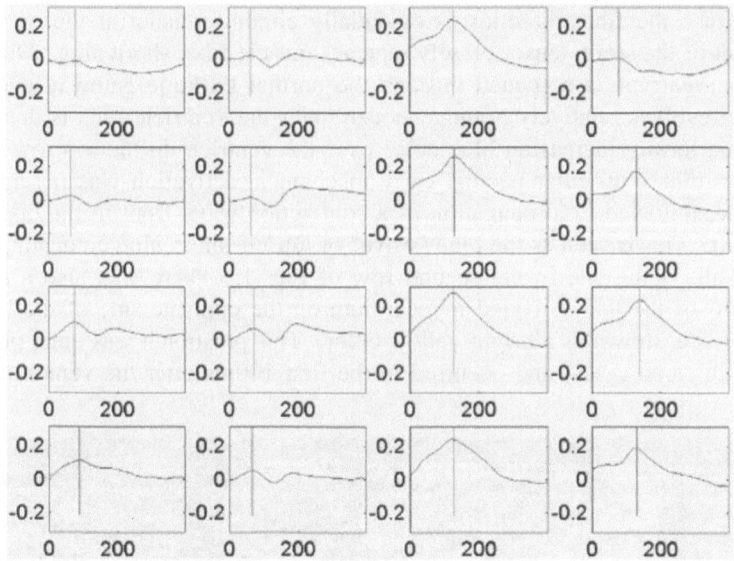

Fig. 2. Each box represents the circumferencial strain vs. time over a 400 ms time period during prestretch and contraction. The top row is the base of the heart, the bottom is the apical region. The columns represent (from left to right) septum, anterior wall, lateral wall and inferior wall. The red vertical bar represents the "mechanical activation time" for each location during RV pacing.

The mechanical data described above can be obtained from a dog in vivo while nearly simultaneously measuring epicardial electrical excitation maps with an electrode array placed around the heart. (The electrical recordings are obtained between MRI image acquisitions.) From these data, maps of both mechanical activation (time of onset of shortening) and electrical activation (time of maximum negative slope in unipolar recordings) were computed. Voltage vs. time plots for the same locations as shown in the Ecc plots of Fig. 2 are shown in Fig 3.

4 Fiber Angle Measurement and Modelling

Fig. 4a and b show maps of fiber orientation for the heart measured in vitro with diffusion tensor imaging. These measurements are made after fixation in order to achieve very high resolution (0.7 × 0.7 × 0.9 mm voxels) using long imaging times (days). The diffusion of water in the muscle was sampled with diffusion encodings oriented in 28 different directions, each of which had a diffusion length of ~700nm. The map shows a clear transmural gradient in fiber angle from the epicardium to the endocardium. The raw fiber angle data can be used to feed a finite element model to describe a smooth field of fiber angles over the heart as shown in Fig. 4b. After the computation of the principle directions of diffusion each eigenvector is projected to the surface to compute fiber angles. These fiber angles are fitted to bilinear hermite

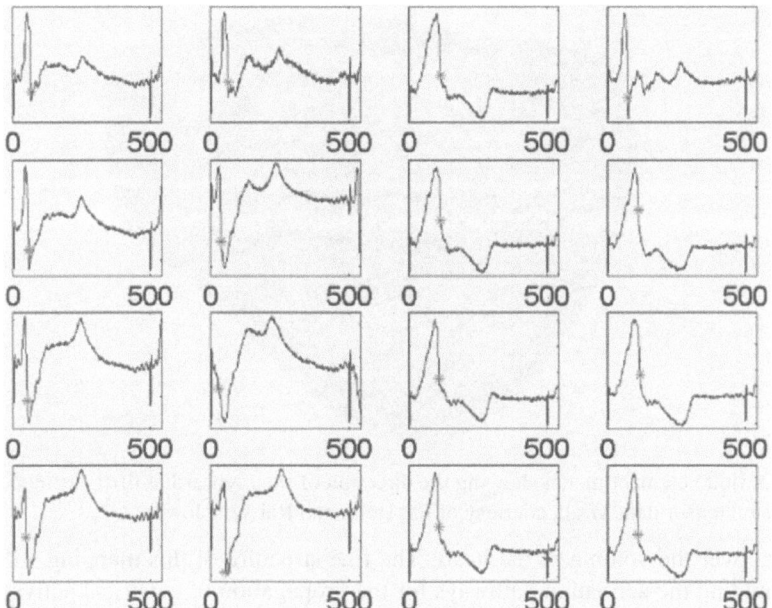

Fig. 3. Unipolar voltage measurements taken from the surface of the heart with a sock electrode. The locations are the same as those shown in Figure 2. The red asterisk represents the time chosen as "electrical activation time" during RV pacing.

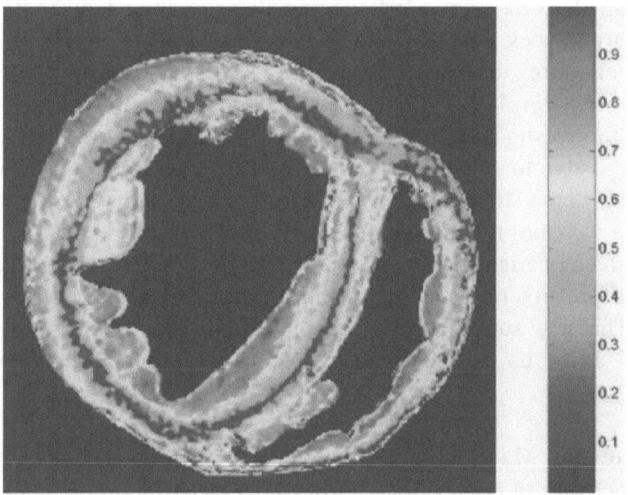

Fig. 4a. A "fiber angle map" in a short axis plane. The color represents the z component of the principal eigen-vector from the diffusion tensor at each location. Blue means the vector is in the plane, red means the vector is orthogonal to the plane. (Data courtesy of Pat Helm and Rai Winslow)

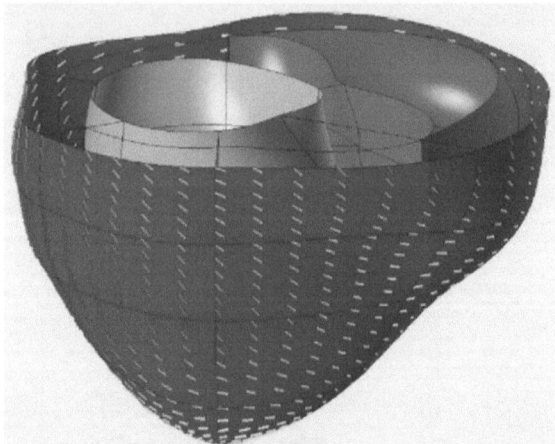

Fig. 4b. A finite element model showing the direction of the myocardial fibers as modeled from the diffusion tensor data. (Data courtesy of Pat Helm and Rai Winslow)

functions over the volume of the heart. The fine structure of this mapping will be key in determining the activation pathways for the propagation of electrical activation, and it may also have a bearing on the mechanical performance of the tissue.

5 Discussion

Strain imaging derived from MRI tagging data combined with electrical mapping using an electrode sock now gives us a new tool for studying the relationship of the temporal kinetics of the electrical and mechanical function during myocardial contraction. High resolution, co-registered fiber angle maps in the same heart will also allow us to investigate the underlying architectural substrate of this function.

It is now possible to study the effect of mechanical stretch on the electrical nature of the heart in vivo. It has been demonstrated that rapid prestretch will stimulate depolarization of the myocardium especially in regions that have the greatest compliance and experience greater relative stretch [5], and that the timing of the application of prestretch determines if an arrhythmic depolarization of the LV will occur [16]. This new strain imaging technique combined with simultaneous electrical mapping will allow us to investigate the local prestretch needed to generate these arrhythmic beats.

Acknowledgments. Many of the results and conclusions reported here are from the collaborative efforts of the Cardiac MRI Research Group at Johns Hopkins and the Medical Imaging Group at NHLBI. The authors would especially like to acknowledge the efforts of Scott Chesnick, Michael Guttman, Chris Moore, Walter O'Dell, Scott Reeder, Frits W. Prinzen, Joni Taylor, Brad Wyman, Joshua Tsitlik, Henry Halperin, Bill Hunter and Elias Zerhouni. The fiber angle mapping is being done as a joint project with Dr. Rai Winslow at JHU. Electrical mapping techniques were taught to us by Bob Lux and Rob McLeod at the CVRTI, University of Utah.

References

1. Axel L and Dougherty L. MR imaging of motion with spatial modulation of magnetization. Radiology 1989; 171: 841-5.
2. Brooks DH and MacLeod RS. Electrical Imaging of the Heart. IEEE Signal Processing Magazine 1997; 14: 24-42.
3. Burnes JE, Taccardi B, and Rudy Y. A noninvasive imaging modality for cardiac arrhythmias. Circulation 2000; 102: 2152-8.
4. Faris O, Evans F, Ozturk C, Ennis D, Taylor J, and McVeigh ER. Correlation Between Electrical and Mechanical Activation in the Paced Canine Heart. International Society of Magnetic Resonance in Medicine: Book of Abstracts 2001.
5. Franz MR, Cima R, Wang D, Profitt D, and Kurz R. Electrophysiological effects of myocardial stretch and mechanical determinants of stretch-activated arrhythmias [published erratum appears in circulation 1992 nov;86(5):1663]. Circulation 1992; 86: 968-78.
6. Garrido L, Wedeen VJ, Kwong KK, Spencer UM, and Kantor HL. Anisotropy of water diffusion in the myocardium of the rat. Circ Res 1994; 74: 789-93.
7. Guttman MA, Prince JL, and McVeigh ER. Tag and contour detection in tagged MR images of the left ventricle. IEEE Trans.Med.Imag. 1994; 13: 74-88.
8. Liu ZW, Jia P, Biblo LA, Taccardi B, and Rudy Y. Endocardial potential mapping from a noncontact nonexpandable catheter: a feasibility study. Ann.Biomed.Eng 1998; 26: 994-1009.
9. MacLeod RS and Brooks DH. Recent progress in inverse problems in electrocardiology. IEEE Eng Med.Biol.Mag. 1998; 17: 73-83.
10. McVeigh ER. MRI of myocardial function: motion tracking techniques. Magn.Reson.Imag. 1996; 14: 137-50.
11. McVeigh ER, Prinzen FW, Wyman BT, Tsitlik JE, Halperin HR, and Hunter WC. Imaging asynchronous mechanical activation of the paced heart with tagged MRI. Magn Reson.Med. 1998; 39: 507-13.
12. Ozturk C and McVeigh ER. Four-dimensional B-spline based motion analysis of tagged MR images: introduction and in vivo validation. Phys.Med.Biol. 2000; 45: 1683-702.
13. Salama G. Optical measurement of transmembrane potential. In: Loew L, ed. Spectroscopic Membrane Probes Vol. III. CRC, Boca Raton. 1988, 137-99.
14. Scollan DF, Holmes A, Winslow R, and FJ. Histological validation of myocardium microstructure obtained from diffusion tensor magnetic resonance imaging. Am J Physiol 1998; 275: H2308-H2318.
15. Wyman BT, Hunter WC, Prinzen FW, and McVeigh ER. Mapping propagation of mechanical activation in the paced heart with MRI tagging. Am.J.Physiol 1999; 276: H881-H891.
16. Zabel M, Koller BS, Sachs F, and Franz MR. Stretch-induced voltage changes in the isolated beating heart: importance of the timing of stretch and implications for stretch-activated ion channels. Cardiovasc.Res. 1996; 32: 120-30.
17. Zerhouni EA, Parish DM, Rogers WJ, Yang A, and Shapiro EP. Human heart: tagging with MR imaging--a method for noninvasive assessment of myocardial motion. Radiology 1988; 169: 59-63.

A 3-D Model-Based Approach for the PET-Functional and MR-Anatomical Cardiac Imaging Data Fusion

Timo Mäkelä[1,2,7], Quoc-Cuong Pham[1], Patrick Clarysse[1],
Jyrki Lötjönen[3], Kirsi Lauerma[4], Helena Hänninen[5,7],
Juhani Knuuti[6], Toivo Katila[2,7], and Isabelle E. Magnin[1]

[1] CREATIS, INSA, Batiment Blaise Pascal, 69621 Villeurbanne Cedex, France
{Quoc-Cuong.Pham, Patrick.Clarysse, Isabelle.Magnin}@creatis.insa-lyon.fr
[2] Laboratory of Biomedical Engineering, Helsinki University of Technology,
P.O.B. 2200, FIN-02015 HUT, Finland
{Timo.Makela, Toivo.Katila}@hut.fi
[3] VTT Information Technology, P.O.Box 1206, FIN-33101 Tampere, Finland
Jyrki.Lotjonen@vtt.fi
[4] Department of Radiology, Helsinki University Central Hospital,
P.O.B. 340, FIN-00029 HUS, Finland
Kirsi.Lauerma@hus.fi
[5] Division of Cardiology, Helsinki University Central Hospital, P.O.B. 340,
FIN-00029 HUS, Finland
Helena.Hanninen@hus.fi
[6] Turku PET Centre, c/o Turku University Central Hospital,
Box 52, FIN-20521, Finland
Juhani.Knuuti@tyks.fi
[7] BioMag Laboratory, Helsinki University Central Hospital, P.O.B. 503,
FIN-00029 HUS, Finland

Abstract. In this paper, an approach for the assessment of 3-D functional maps of the heart is proposed. It relies on the model-based co-registration of MR anatomical and PET metabolic images and the extraction of an individualized anatomical heart model from MR images. This results in a 3-D geometrical model of the heart for which functional parameters such as FDG uptake can be attributed and visualized.

1   Introduction

Cardiac viability studies mainly rely on the integration of the myocardial perfusion, metabolism and contractile function. Metabolism can be analyzed with Positron Emission Tomography (PET) and contractile function can be studied using Magnetic Resonance Imaging (MRI), for instance. In order to assess the cardiac viability assessment, it is crucial to accurately co-register the multi-modality images in order to be able corroborate the complementary functional information. In the "MunichHeart" software, endocardial and epicardial contours are manually delineated in Short Axis (SA) MR images and coregistered

T. Katila et al. (Eds.): FIMH 2001, LNCS 2230, pp. 83–90, 2001.

with the same contours extracted from PET or SPECT (Single Photon Emission Tomography) using the maximum count detection algorithm [1]. In [2], maximal myocardial deformation from tagged MRI and FDG-PET metabolism was combined using fuzzy rules to generate polar maps representing the viability. The registration was performed manually with the help of the long axis angles defined in the MRI protocol. In this paper, we present a model based approach for the automatic registration and segmentation of the right (RV) and left ventricles (LV) of the heart in PET and MR images. It provides a 3-D geometric representation on which functional information can be displayed. The data and the approach are presented in Subsections 2.1 and 2.2, respectively. Results are presented in Section 3 and discussed in Section 4.

2   Material and Method

2.1   Cardiac Imaging Protocol

The data set is composed of MR and PET images of ten patients suffering from three vessels coronary artery disease [3]. Mean age was 69 (8 men, 2 women). All patients underwent MR and fluorine-18-deoxyglucose (FDG) PET imaging within 10 days.

The MR imaging was performed at the Department of Radiology of Helsinki University Central Hospital with a 1.5 T Siemens Magnetom Vision imager (Siemens, Erlangen, Germany). A series of 39 ECG-gated contiguous transaxial images was acquired during free respiration using TurboFLASH sequence (Fig. 1a). The pixel size and the slice thickness were 1.95 x 1.95 mm and 10 mm, respectively. Five ECG-gated breath-hold cine SA sections 15 mm apart were also acquired (Fig. 1b). The pixel size for SA slices was 1.25 x 1.25 mm and slice thickness 7 mm. About 15 time points were taken for each section with the repetition time of 40 msec.

Static PET imaging was performed using a Siemens ECAT (Siemens/CTI, Knoxville, USA) PET scanner. A series of 16 contiguous transmission and emission images was acquired. The pixel size and the slice thickness were 2.41 x 2.41 mm and 6.75 mm, respectively (Fig. 1c, d).

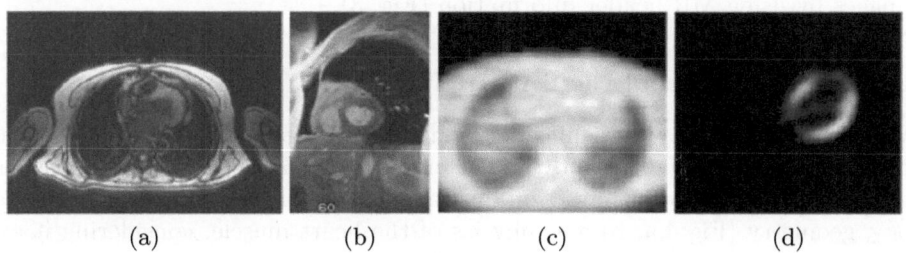

     (a)   (b)   (c)   (d)

Fig. 1. (a) Transaxial and (b) SA MR images, (c) transmission and (d) emission PET images.

2.2 Method Overview

The aim of the overall approach is to extract a 3-D anatomical model of the heart from patient MR images and to incorporate functional data, such as FDG uptake and other clinically relevant parameters to the model. The process is summarized in Fig. 2. First, MR transaxial images are co-registered with the PET transmission image. The obtained registration parameters are used to register transaxial MR images and the PET emission image. PET images that corresponds SA MR images are calculated by using MR header information. Then, a 3-D biventricular model is initialized in the SA MR images to segment the myocardium. The deformed model is finally transformed into the registered SA PET image to obtain FDG uptake values. The main steps of the method are summarized in the following sections.

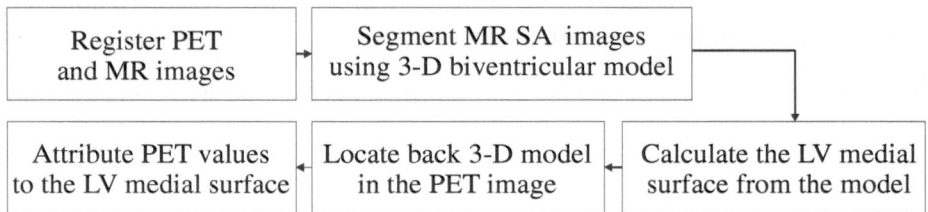

Fig. 2. Extraction of the 3-D anatomical and functional model of the heart including PET-FDG uptake : main steps of the process.

2.3 PET-MR Image Registration

The method for registration of MR and PET images is fully described in [4] and [5]. It minimizes the distance between the point set from segmented PET transmission image surfaces and a distance map [6] built upon the segmented transaxial MR surfaces. The thorax and lungs surfaces are segmented from transaxial MR and transmission PET images by using the deformable model based segmentation method presented in [7]. SA PET slices are computed from registered images by using MR header information (Fig. 3).

2.4 Segmentation of the SA MR Images

We use a 3-D prior biventricular deformable model of the myocardium to simultaneously segment the LV and the RV in SA MR images. In order to constrain the segmentation, we introduce in our model a priori information about topology, geometry (Fig 4.a, b) and physics of the heart muscle, considering it as a linear elastic medium.

First, the template is manually initialized in the MR volume (Fig 5.). Then it is submitted to a force field derived from the image and elastically deformed

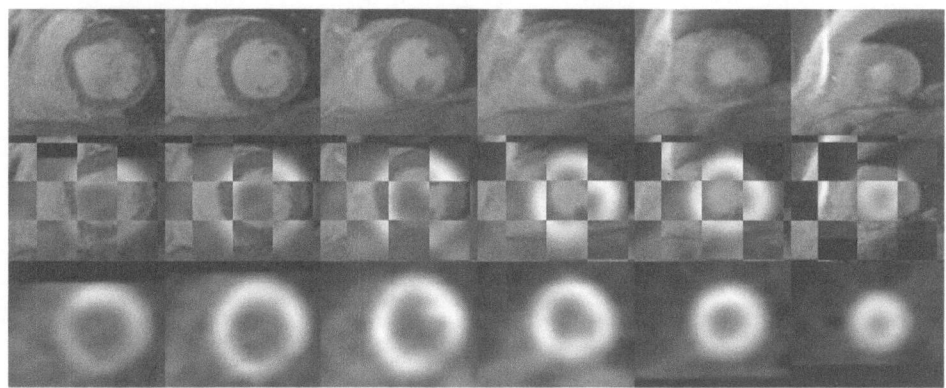

Fig. 3. The 2-D representation of registered (computed) end-diastolic SA MR (top) and PET emission (bottom) image slices for the H1 case. In the middle row, the images are overlaid in block format to visualize registration results.

until its boundaries fit the contours extracted from the data. We thus obtain a 3-D geometrical representation of the patient's heart. Fig. 6 shows segmentation results obtained for 2 patients. This approach has been fully described in [8].

2.5   Extracting Functional Data Associated to the Model

Functional data can be attributed to the cells and nodes of the 3-D biventricular model. Some parameters with clinical interest can be derived from MR Imaging. First, the model is labeled so that it is possible to directly separate the right and left ventricles or obtain internal and external surfaces. Moreover, cavity volumes, myocardial mass and local wall thickness are computed. In order to enrich the model with metabolic information the model is transformed into the registered PET-FDG emission image. Medial surface is automatically calculated between LV endo- and epicardial surfaces. The medial surface nodes, M_i, are calculated as follows. For each node A_i, of the endocardial surface, we compute the normal to the surface that intersects the epicardial surface at B_i. M_i is taken as the middle point of the line $[A_i B_i]$ (Fig. 7a). Surfaces are transformed to registered PET emission image and a FDG uptake mean value is computed at each surface node of the medial surface (Fig. 7b, middle contour) in a 5 x 5 x 5 neighborhood (Fig. 7c).

3   Displays of 3-D Functional Maps

Fig. 8 a,b illustrate the FDG metabolic activity over the LV medial surface for 2 cases. Right ventricular and epicardial surfaces are shown in transparency. Visualizations are performed using the VTK software library [9].

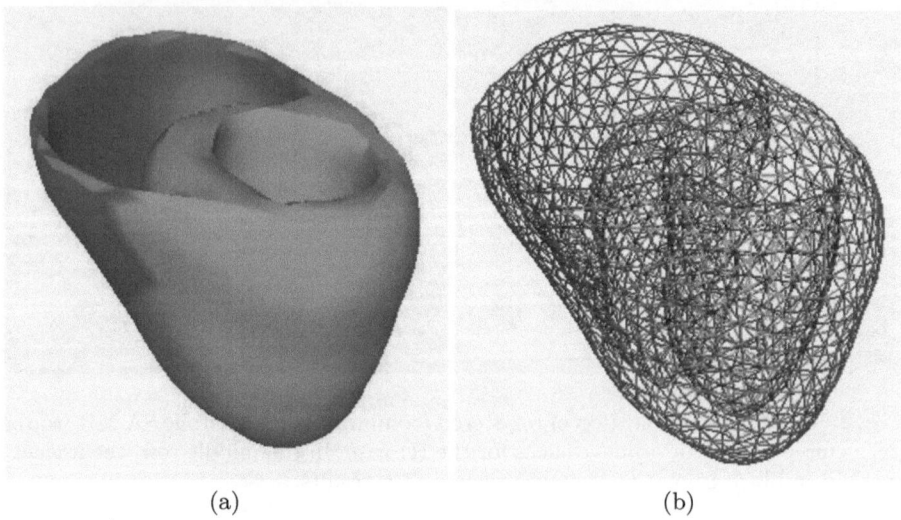

(a)   (b)

Fig. 4. (a) 3-D prior biventricular model, (b) Corresponding mesh (1853 nodes, 7257 elements).

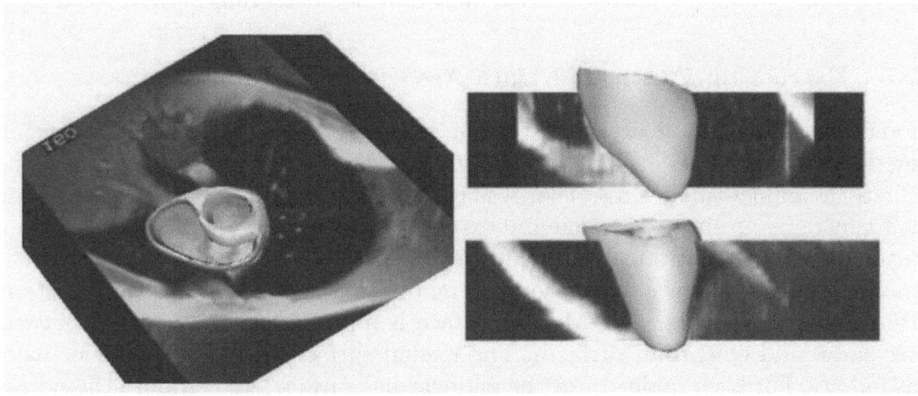

Fig. 5. Model immersed in SA MR images.

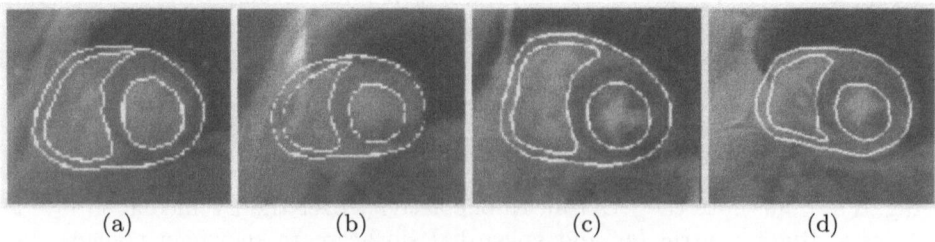

(a)   (b)   (c)   (d)

Fig. 6. Segmentation results of basal (BS) and mid-ventricular (MV) slice of (a) patient H1 (BS), (b) patient H1 (MV), (c) patient H2 (BS) and (d) patient H2 (MV).

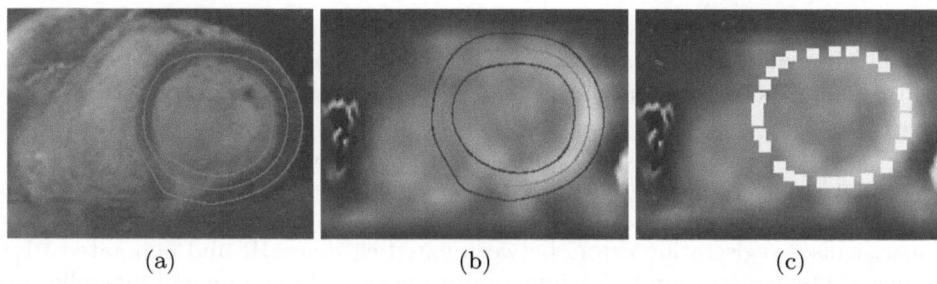

(a)   (b)   (c)

Fig. 7. (a) Intersection of endocardial (intrinsic contour), epicardial (outermost con-
~~~~) the
con-
edial

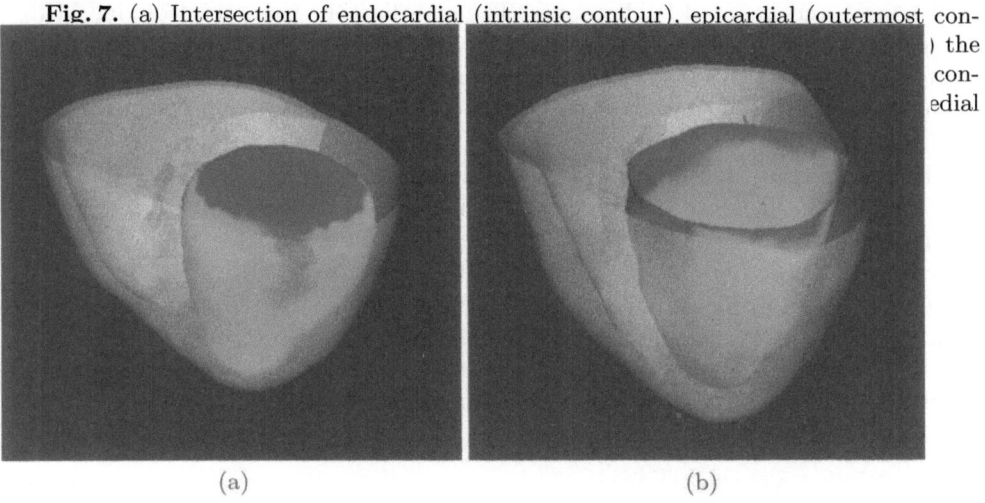

(a)   (b)

(a)   (b)

Fig. 8. 3-D representation of the FDG PET uptake values of (a) patient H1 and (b) patient H2.

4   Discussion and Conclusion

Using the described imaging protocol, we are able to combine MR anatomical and PET functional data for the same heart. The reliability of the result mainly depends on the accuracy of the PET-MRI registration. Visually satisfactory results were obtained with 9 over the 10 available cases. For one bad case, there was unexpected artifacts in FDG PET data. Two of the good biventricular deformable model results were illustrated in this paper. For some of the cases, slight manual intervention to move medial surface in PET image was needed. For better validation of the method phantom experiments or simulated images will be needed.

In [5], we have proposed a quantification of the registration accuracy based on a distance between segmented surfaces. Transaxial MR images were obtained with a snapshot technique during free respiration. In comparison, PET transmission images could be considered as an integral image over the acquisition time (about 10 minutes). This might lead to differences in the thorax shape and diaphragm position between these two imaging methods and causes error in this surface based registration method. Also twisting and contraction of the heart causes registration errors between gated cardiac MR and non-gated PET images. The registration of SA images was performed between end-diastolic cine MR images and ungated PET images. The end-diastolic time point of cine MR images was selected, because ungated PET images result from the uptake integration over several heart cycle and mostly represent the diastolic phase. We are going to investigate the accurate validation of the registration approach through image simulations.

In the segmentation procedure, the initialization step is crucial. We are currently working on its automation. As the model is locally deformed, it has to be positioned quite close to the contours. This could be achieved by a rigid registration method (Iterative Closest Point [10] for example).

One can also propose different alternative strategies to attribute PET-FDG uptake values to the model. This concerns our future work. We believe that the 3-D functional maps proposed in this paper are valuable tools to help the cardiologist in the interpretation of multi-modality cardiac imaging data for the better diagnosis of the myocardial viability.

Acknowledgments. This study was partly granted by the Scientific Department of the French Embassy in Finland, the Region Rhône Alpes, through the ADéMO project, the Finnish Cultural Foundation and Tekniikan edistämissäätiö.

References

1. Nekolla S., Miethaner C., Nguyen N., Ziegler S., Schwaiger M. Reproducibility of polar map generation and assessment of defect severity and extent assessment in myocardial perfusion imaging using positron emission tomography. Eur J Nuvl Med **25** (1998) 1313–1321.
2. Behloul F., Janier M., Croisille P., Poirier C., Boudraa A., Unterreiner R., Mason J., Revel D. Automatic assessment of myocardial viability based on PET-MRI data fusion. Proceedings of the 20th annual international conference of the IEEE Engineering in Medicine and Biology Society, **1** (1998) 429–495.
3. Lauerma K., Niemi P., Hänninen H., Janatuinen T., Voipio-Pulkki L., Knuuti J., Toivonen L., Mäkelä T., Mäkijärvi M. A. , Aronen H. J.: Multimodality MR imaging assessment of myocardial viability: combination of first-pass and late contrast enhancement to wall motion dynamics and comparison with FDG-PET. Radiology, **217** (2000) 729–736.

4. Mäkelä T., Clarysse P., Lötjönen J., Sipilä O., Hänninen H., Nenonen J., Lauerma K., Knuuti J., Katila T. and Magnin I. E.: A method for registration of cardiac MR and PET images for the myocardial viability study. In: Marzullo, P. (ed.): NATO advanced research workshop - Understanding Cardiac Imaging Techniques From Basic Pathology to Image Fusion. NATO Science Series: Life and Behavioural Sciences. IOS Press **332** (2001) 155–165.
5. Mäkelä T., Clarysse P., Lötjönen J., Sipilä O., Hänninen H., Nenonen J., Lauerma K., Knuuti J., Katila T. and Magnin I. E.: A new method for the registration of cardiac MR and PET images using deformable model based segmentation of the main thorax structures. MICCAI 2001. Accepted.
6. Borgefors G.: Hierarchical chamfer matching: A parametric edge matching algorithm. IEEE Trans. Pattern Anal. Machine Intell., **6** (1988) 849–865.
7. Lötjönen J., Reissman P.-J., Magnin I.E. and Katila T.: Model extraction from magnetic resonance volume data using the deformable pyramid. Medical Image Analysis, **4** (1999) 387–406.
8. Pham Q.C., Vincent F., Clarysse P., Croisille P., Magnin I.E.: A FEM-Based deformable model for the 3D segmentation and tracking of the Heart in Cardiac MRI. ISPA 2001. Accepted.
9. Homepage of The Visualization ToolKit (VTK), www.kitware.com.
10. Besl P.J. and McKay N.D.: A method for regisration of 3-D shapes. IEEE Trans. Pattern Anal. Machine Intell., **14** (1992) 239–256.

3D Regularisation and Segmentation of Factor Volumes to Process PET H₂¹⁵O Myocardial Perfusion Studies

Frédérique Frouin[1], Paté Boubacar[1], Vincent Frouin[2], Alain De Cesare[1], Andrew Todd-Pokropek[1,3], Pascal Merlet[4], and Alain Herment[1]

[1] U494 INSERM CHU Pitié-Salpêtrière, F-75634 Paris cedex 13, France
Frederique.Frouin@imed.jussieu.fr,
WWW home page: http://www.imed.jussieu.fr
[2] Service Hospitalier Frédéric Joliot, Direction des Sciences du Vivant, Commissariat à l'Energie Atomique, 4 place du Général Leclerc F-91400 Orsay, France
[3] Departement of Medical Physics and Bioengineering, University College of London, Gower Street, London, WC1E 6BT, UK
[4] Service de Médecine Nucléaire, Hôpital Henri Mondor, F-94000 Créteil, France

Abstract. A 3D image processing method to increase reproducibility in the handling of PET myocardial perfusion studies is proposed. It is based on the 3D regularization of factor volumes, which are estimated by FAMIS (Factor Analysis of Medical Image Sequences). The resulting regularized factor volumes correspond to right and left cavities and to perfused tissues. They are then submitted to a C-means classification, looking for 4 clusters. Some rules of connectivity are applied to the resulting clusters to achieve the segmentation of heart cavities and myocardium. Thereafter, kinetics in the left ventricle and in the myocardium can be computed from the previously determined volumes of interest, and myocardial blood flow (MBF) is estimated by a conventional compartmental analysis.

1 Introduction

PET myocardial perfusion studies are primordial when absolute quantitation of myocardial blood flow is required [1]. Oxygen-15 labeled water (H₂¹⁵O) studies offer a large potential interest, since water is an ideal tracer to study perfusion. The short half-life of oxygen-15 allows to repeat experiments in a short time, which is useful to study rest and stress conditions, for instance. However, the signal to noise ratio (SNR) of these studies is very low. That is the reason why some additional scans (using C¹⁵O or ¹⁸FDG) are needed to delineate the myocardium [2]. This has hindered the generalisation of such studies in a clinical context. To overcome this limitation, some *a posteriori* image processing methods have recently been proposed. They are mainly based on statistical data analysis [3], and more particularly on factor analysis methods, such as Factor Analysis of Medical Image Sequences (FAMIS)[4],[5] . In case of a first-pass myocardial perfusion study, FAMIS can synthesise a whole dynamic series into 3 or 4 kinetics

T. Katila et al. (Eds.): FIMH 2001, LNCS 2230, pp. 91–96, 2001.

(called factors) and associated images (called factor images), which correspond to 1) right cavities, 2) possibly lungs, 3) left cavities and 4) myocardium and other perfused tissues. FAMIS algorithm consists first of estimating factors, then of computing factor images from raw data and factors, using a conventional least-squares method. The quality of factor images strongly depends on the noise level present in the raw data [6]. We have proposed a 2D regularisation of factor images [7] to improve the quality of factor images in case of raw studies with a low SNR. Its principle is to add some neighbourhood constraints in the reconstruction of the factor images, and so to improve the quality of factor images, especially regarding the SNR. The method has proved to be useful in the processing of $H_2{}^{15}O$ myocardial studies [4]. The first applications were carried out on exams acquired with a multi-slice PET scanner. However the method does not take into account the features of up-to-date PET scanners, which provide data with a nearly 3D isotropic resolution. Moreover, with up to 63 slices, the data volume to be processed becomes huge and manual contouring of volumes of interest is a complex and fastidious task.

This paper describes the developments that we propose to better process 3D data. Firstly, the generalization of the regularization method to 3D data is described. Secondly, a method for the automatic contouring of heart cavities and myocardium is proposed. The processing chain is illustrated on a clinical study. The potential interest of the method is discussed and possible applications in other modalities are proposed.

2   Materials and Methods

2.1   Materials: Dynamic Perfusion Studies

Dynamic studies were acquired with an ECAT HR+ PET scanner, according to the protocol given in [2]. The injected dose was lowered to take into account the sensitivity of the PET scanner. The acquisition was performed in 2D mode, i.e. with the septa. For each time, volumes were reconstructed using a standard FBP algorithm. Four dimensional data sets (three space dimensions plus time) were finally obtained.

2.2   FAMIS Algorithm

The FAMIS algorithm was extended to process 4D data sets, as described in [8]. Its consists in reducing the data set $S(v,t)$, where v represents the voxel variable and t the time variable, to a limited number, N_k, of factors, $C_k(t)$, and of associated factor volumes, $D_k(v)$, according to the equation :

$$S(v,t) = \sum_{k=1}^{N_k} C_k(t).D_k(v) + e(v,t). \tag{1}$$

The term $e(v,t)$ is the error term associated to each voxel at a specified time. The error is assumed to be zero-mean, and its covariance matrix is assumed to be known. Positivity constraints are applied to both $C_k(t)$ and $D_k(v)$ terms, in order to be consistent with a physiological interpretation.

Once the factors $C_k(t)$ are estimated, the conventional estimation of the factor volumes $D_k(v)$ is based on the minimisation of the term E_1 :

$$E_1 = \sum_{t=1}^{N_t} \sum_{v=1}^{N_v} e(v,t)^2, \tag{2}$$

$$= \sum_{t=1}^{N_t} \sum_{v=1}^{N_v} \left(S(v,t) - \sum_{k=1}^{N_k} C_k(t).D_k(v) \right)^2. \tag{3}$$

Finally, the contribution c_k of the kth couple of factor and factor volume is computed according to the equation :

$$c_k = \frac{\sum_1^{N_t} \sum_1^{N_v} C_k(t).D_k(v)}{\sum_1^{N_k} \sum_1^{N_t} \sum_1^{N_v} C_k(t).D_k(v)}. \tag{4}$$

2.3   3D Regularisation of Factor Volumes

The goal of the regularisation is to improve the quality of factor images, by introducing some *a priori* knowledge in their construction. The conventional way consists of setting some similarity constraints between neighbouring voxels, which has for mathematical formalism:

$$E_{2k} = \sum_{v=1}^{N_v} \sum_{v^*=1}^{N_{nv}} h_\alpha(D_k(v^*), D_k(v)), \tag{5}$$

where N_{nv} is the number of voxels, which are connected to the voxel v. Practically, the six-connectivity is chosen: it is sufficient to introduce the neighbouring constraints and it enables us to reduce the number of computations which are required by the 26-connectivity. The h_α function is the Hubert function: it is quadratic for small differences in image intensity and linear elsewhere.

Let x be $(D_k(v^*) - D_k(v))$, $h_\alpha(x) = \begin{cases} x^2 & \text{for } -\alpha \le x \le \alpha \\ \alpha(2x - \alpha) & \text{for } x > \alpha \\ -\alpha(2x + \alpha) & \text{for } x < -\alpha \end{cases}$.

The regularised factor volumes $D_k(v)$ are estimated by minimising the term E:

$$E = E_1 + \mu.\sum_{k=1}^{N_k} \frac{1}{c_k} E_{2k} \tag{6}$$

where μ is a positive coefficient which sets the trade-off between the fit to the raw data and the *a priori* of smoothness in the factor volumes.

2.4   3D Classification and Segmentation of Heart Cavities and Myocardium

A N_k component vector $\left(\frac{D_1(v^*)}{Max_v(D_1(v))}, \frac{D_2(v^*)}{Max_v(D_2(v))}, ..., \frac{D_{N_k}(v^*)}{Max_v(D_{N_k}(v))} \right)$ is associated to each voxel v^*. These N_v vectors are submitted to a C-means algorithm. When $N_k = 3$, clusters are initialised by the four following vectors $(1, 0, 0)$, $(0, 1, 0)$, $(0, 0, 1)$, and $(0.1, 0.1, 0.1)$. The resulting clusters are functional clusters and they do not match the anatomic regions. For instance, myocardial and hepatic tissues are in the same cluster, since their functional behaviour is nearly the same in a perfusion study. To separate such functional structures, some further post-processing has to be applied to 3D clusters. The largest 3D connected volumes are first isolated. Then left cavities are separated from large vessels, such as the aorta. In a last step, a simple *a priori* geometrical knowledge is introduced to define myocardial tissue: myocardium is defined as tissue surrounding the left ventricle. A 3D spatial contiguity constraint is applied which ensures that the maximal distance between one myocardial voxel and one left ventricular voxel should be less than 4 voxels.

3   Results

For first-pass myocardial perfusion studies, FAMIS estimates generally three structures, which can be identified to right cavities, left cavities, and perfused tissues, which are mainly the myocardial and hepatic tissues in the field-of-view of the exam.. Figure 1 shows the regularised factor volumes which have been estimated using $\alpha = \frac{Max(D_k(v))}{100}$ and $\mu = 0.25$. The term E is minimised by the Flechter-Reeves's algorithm. Convergence is generally obtained after 20 iterations.

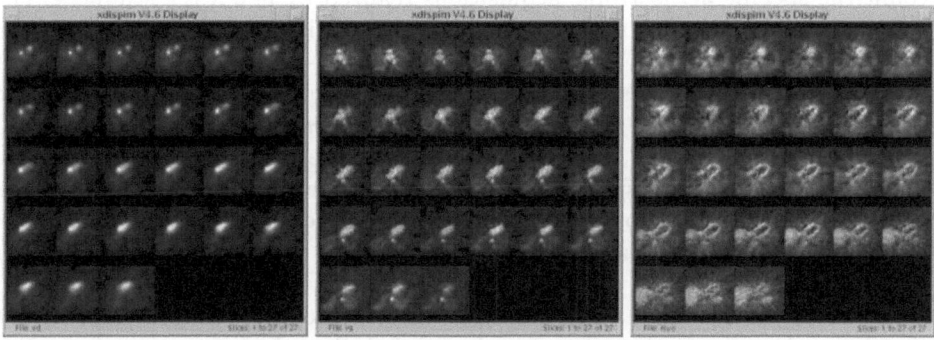

Fig. 1. Regularised factor volumes (27 consecutive slices) estimated by FAMIS software. From left to right : right cavities, left cavities, and myocardium plus other perfused tissues, such as liver.

The C-means classification identifies 4 clusters, which are defined as 1) right cavities, 2) left cavities, 3) myocardium and other perfused tissues, and 4) background and lungs. The further processing of clusters which is based on geometrical considerations provides the segmentation which is shown by Figure 2.

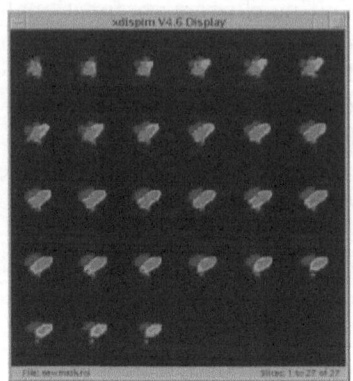 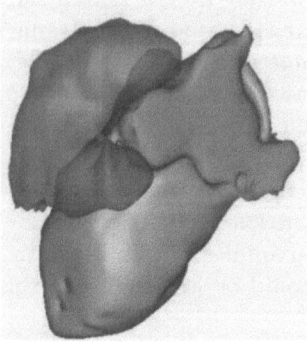

Fig. 2. Results of the segmentation on the 27 consecutive slices. Surface view of segmented structures generated by the Anatomist software (SHFJ, CEA). Right cavities are in blue colour, left cavities in red colour and myocardium is in light maroon colour.

4   Discussion

The interest of the regularisation of factor images has already been demonstrated [7]. The generalisation of the method to 3D data is necessary to take into account the specific 3D isotropic acquisitions realized by new PET scanners. The classification is a way to segment the different cardiac structures based on the regularised factor images or factor volumes. The C-means algorithm is robust when an adequate initialisation is performed. In our case, this initialisation can be easily performed, since the clusters can be *a priori* defined : right cavities and left cavities, myocardium, and background. In some cases, it may be useful to add a fifth cluster, corresponding to lungs and which can be initialised by the (0, 0.3, 0.3) vector. Compared to threshold-based methods, which need *a priori* calibration, our method is more simple to adapt to different cameras. Another interest of the method is that it takes into account the functional information which is in the dynamic first-pass data. As a consequence, right cavities, left cavities and perfused tissues can be isolated during the same procedure. The knowledge of the left ventricular position is useful to segment the myocardium. Thereafter, the geometrical constraint which has been introduced to position the myocardium is sufficient to separate the myocardium from the liver. The potential applications of this segmentation are not restricted to $H_2{}^{15}O$ studies.

It could be applied to ^{13}NH$_3$ PET studies, which are largely used for assessing myocardial perfusion. Moreover, some applications of this principle have been tested on MR first-pass perfusion studies. The goal of the proposed segmentation is not to solve the partial volume effect : some more precise *a priori* information would then be necessary to take it into account. Our recommandation is that the contamination of myocardium by the left cavity has to be taken into account by the compartmental model, as it is done when manual segmentation is performed. The limits of the algorithm in case of the different pathologies, which introduce a reduction of MBF, should be defined.

5   Conclusion

An automatic method to segment first-pass myocardial perfusion studies has been proposed. It takes advantage of the presence in the same study of heart cavities and myocardium. Although the different structures are not well separated on raw data, the processing based on factor analysis and followed by a classification allows us to separate them. The method needs no *a priori* calibration and its principle can be applied to a large variety of first-pass myocardial studies.

References

1. Bergmann S.R.: Clinical applications of myocardial perfusion assessments made with oxygen-15 water and positron emission tomography. Cardiology **88** (1997) 71–79.
2. Merlet P., Mazoyer B., Hittinger L. et al.: Assessment of coronary reserve in man: comparison between positron emission tomography with oxygen-15-labeled water and intracoronary Doppler technique. J. Nucl. Med. **34** (1993) 1899–1904.
3. Hermansen F., Ashburner J., Spinks T., Kooner J., Camici P., Lammersta A.: Generation of myocardial factor images directly from the dynamic oxygen-15-water scan without use of an oxygen-15-carbon monoxyde blood-pool scan. J. Nucl. Med. **39** (1998) 1696–1702.
4. Bouchareb Y., Frouin, F., De Cesare A., Merlet P., Frouin V., Gregoire M.C., Herment A.: Régularisation de l'Analyse Factorielle des Séquences d'Images Médicales (AFSIM). Application aux études de perfusion myocardique à l'eau marquée en TEP. Innov. Techn. Biol. Med. **20** (1999) 93–100.
5. Ahn J., Lee D., Lee J., Kim S., Cheon G., Yeo J., Shin S., Chung J., Lee, M.: Quantification of regional myocardial blood flow using dynamic H$_2^{15}$O PET and factor analysis. J. Nucl. Med. **42** (2001) 782-787.
6. Buvat I., Benali H., Di Paola R.: Statistical distribution of factors and factor images in factor analysis of medical image sequences Phys. Med. Biol. **43** (1998) 421–434.
7. Frouin F., De Cesare A., Bouchareb, Y., Todd-Pokropek A., Herment, A.: Spatial regularization applied to factor analysis of medical image sequences. Phys. Med. Biol. **44** (1999) 2289–2306.
8. Frouin F., Cinotti L., Benali H. et al.: Extraction of functional volumes from medical dynamic volumetric data sets. Comput. Med. Imaging Graph. **17** (1993) 397–404.

In Vivo Assessment of Rat Hearts with and without Myocardial Infarction by Cine NMR – Comparison of the NMR Method to Invasive Techniques and Application to Intervention Studies

M. Nahrendorf[1], K.-H. Hiller[1], K. Hu[2], C. Waller[2], F. Wiesmann[2], J. Ruff[1], G. Ertl[2], A. Haase[1], and W.R. Bauer[2]

[1]Physikalisches Institut (EP5), Universität Würzburg, Am Hubland, 97074 Würzburg
[2]Medizinische Universitätsklinik Würzburg, Josef Schneider Str. 2, 97080 Würzburg, Germany

Abstract. Aim of the study was to test the feasibility of cine-NMR for assessment of the infarcted rat heart and to compare the results to established methods. Thereafter, the value of cine-NMR was tested in studies investigating interventions to change the course of the remodeling process. NMR was performed for determination of left ventricular (LV) volumes and mass, MI-size and cardiac output. After MRI rats underwent conventional hemodynamic measurements for determination of cardiac output and LV volumes by electromagnetic flowmeter and pressure-volume curves. LV wet weight was determined. MI-size was determined by histology. MRI-acquired MI-size ($18.5 \pm 2\%$) was smaller than histology ($22.8 \pm 2.5\%$, $p < 0.05$) with close correlation ($r = 0.97$). There was agreement in LV mass between MRI and wet weight ($r = 0.97$, $p < 0.05$) and in the MRI- and flowmeter measurements of cardiac output ($r = 0.80$, $p < 0.05$). Volume by MRI differed from pressure-volume curves with good correlation ($r = 0.96$, $p < 0.05$). In conclusion, cine-NMR is a valuable diagnostic tool applicable to the rat model of MI. Being non-invasive and exact it offers new insights in the remodeling process after MI because serial measurements are possible.

1 Introduction

The rat heart infarct model has proved to be predictive for cardiac remodeling after myocardial infarction (MI) in patients and for therapy [1]. Being noninvasive and exact nuclear magnetic resonance (NMR) can offer new insights allowing serial investigations of rat cardiac morphology and function. Aim of the study was a comparison of data acquired by NMR and conventional, established methods [2, 3]. After completion of the validation experiments the technique was applied to several interventional studies in the rat heart infarction model, as impact of transmyocardial laser revascularisation on remodeling after MI, influence of androgene levels on post infarct remodeling and influence of a cerivastatin therapy on left ventricular remodeling.

2 Methods

In group A 8 controls and 8 rats 16 weeks after myocardial infarction (MI) were investigated on a 7 T-Biospec (Bruker, Germany) using an ECG-triggered Cine-FLASH-sequence. A home built rat size whole body coil was used as transmitter and

T. Katila et al. (Eds.): FIMH 2001, LNCS 2230, pp. 97-103, 2001.
© Springer-Verlag Berlin Heidelberg 2001

a surface coil as receiver. For imaging, we used an ECG-triggered fast gradient echo (FLASH) cine sequence [4]. Flip angle was 30 to 40°, echo time was 1.1 ms, repetition time 3.2 ms. 12 frames per heart cycle were obtained. The total acquisition time (TAT) for one cine sequence was 40 to 50 s depending on heart rate (TAT=128 phase encoding steps * 2 averaging steps * length of one heart cycle). The measurements were averaged four times to increase signal to noise ratio. 15 to 18 contiguous ventricular short axis slices of 1 mm thickness were acquired to cover the entire heart. Total scan time was in the range of 15 min. With a field of view of 3 to 4 cm and an image matrix of 128 by 128 in plane resolution was 230 to 310 μm. Data analysis was done using an operator-interactive threshold technique. Myocardial and ventricular slice volumes were determined from end-diastolic and end-systolic images by multiplication of compartment area and slice thickness (1mm). Total volumes were calculated as sum of all slices. Left ventricular mass was calculated as LV myocardial volume multiplied by the myocardial specific gravity (1.05 g/cm^3). Myocardial infarct size (MI-size) was determined for every slice as the myocardial portion with significant thinning and akinesia or dyskinesia during systole. MI-size was calculated by dividing the sum of the endocardial and epicardial circumferences occupied by the infarct by the sum of the total epicardial and endocardial circumferences of the left ventricle. This method was adapted from the histological determination of MI-size first described by Pfeffer et al. [2].

After NMR hemodynamic measurements were performed for determination of the same parameters by electromagnetic flowmeter and postmortal pressure-volume curves (simultaneous infusion at 0.76ml/min and pressure recording, end-diastolic volume is infused volume at in vivo measured end-diastolic pressure) [2, 3]. The left ventricles were weighted. In group B NMR-acquired and histological MI-size (picric red dye after formalin fixation) [2] were compared in 26 rats.

3 Results

As shown in the table, good correlation between NMR and invasive techniques was found. Significant differences between methods were detected in infarct size, end-diastolic volume and ejection fraction.

	NMR		conventional method		r
MI-size %	18.5±2		22.8±2.5*		r=0.97
	MI	control	MI	control	
LV mass (mg)	865.1±39.2	537.6±19.6	865.1±41.3	540.3±18.4	r=0.97
EDV (μl)	737.0±70.5	343.9±8.4	671.1±64.1*	262.7±12.8*	r=0.96
SV (μl)	259.1±10.4	224.4±7.8	245.8±13.5	221.2±9.2	r=0.70
EF (%)	36.7±2.4	65.3±1.6	41.9±3.8*	84.4±2.3*	r=0.97

Data is given in mean±SEM. r: correlation coefficient of methods (MI plus control), * $p < 0.05$ vs. NMR of the same group, EDV: end-diastolic volume, SV: stroke volume.

5 Conclusion

The study showed good agreement of NMR-acquired data with established methods for LV mass and stroke volume. With a difference of 5% both methods of MI-size determination correlate well. The difference to the NMR-method is due to inhomogeneity of shrinkage caused by formalin fixation of the excised hearts. There was good correlation of postmortal determined to in vivo measured end-diastolic volume. The significant difference was bigger in the controls than in MI-rats (23.4% and 9.0%) and is attributed to the absence of enregy dependent, active relaxation in hearts arrested by potassium chloride. In conclusion, application of NMR to the rat model of myocardial infarction is promising to shed new light on the pathomechanisms of cardiac remodeling, because changes during this process can be monitored in intact individual animals. Serial characterisation of infarct size allows investigation of ongoing changes of the MI-scar.

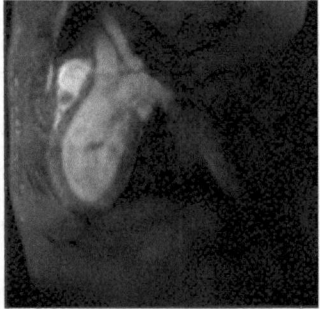

Fig.1. Diastolic long axis frame of control rat. This is one of twelve frames covering the cardiac cycle (average length in the rat 300 ms), which can be animated as a movie. Image shows left ventricle with inflow and outflow tract.

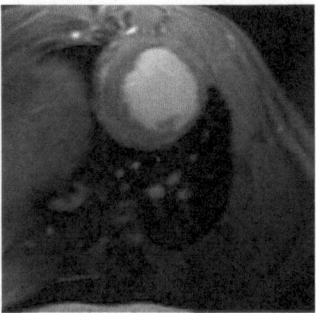

Fig.2. Systolic short axis frame of rat 12 weeks after anterolateral myocardial infarction. Infarcted region has lost its function and is characterized by a thinned wall.

4 Application Studies

4.1 Transmyocardial Laser Revascularisation Improves Perfusion but Enhances Left Ventricular Remodeling in Rats after Myocardial Infarction

Hypertrophy following MI causes diffuse hypoperfusion of the remote myocardium. We therefore used the MI rat model for assessment of transmyocardial laser revascularisation (TMLR). 8 weeks after coronary artery ligation rats had Cine-NMR, thereafter TMLR was done. A selfdesigned Holmium:Yag laser system emitting a wavelength at 2.1μm (pulse energy 4J, pulse duration 1 ms, 365μm fiber diameter) was placed in soft contact to the remote myocardium. 4 weeks after TMLR a second Cine-NMR including dobutamine-stress (10 μl/kg/min via tail vein) was follwed by high resolution spin labeling perfusion imaging (pixel size 140 μm). For assessment of perfusion changes induced by TMLR treatment, spin-labeling MRI was performed as described previously [5] in a 11.75 Tesla wide bore magnet (AMX 500, Bruker, Karlsruhe, FRG). The principle of the measurement is that spins of a selected imaging slice are inverted and T_1 relaxation of these spins towards equilibrium is observed. Due to perfusion non-inverted (equilibrium) spins flow into the slice. This results in a decrease of the apparent proton relaxation time in tissue. Perfusion imaging was performed in isolated retrogradely perfused hearts obtained from rats of the TMLR group (n=10).

TMLR-areas were located by corresponding H&E histology. TLMR-areas were better perfused (3.89 ± 0.83ml/min/g at rest and 2.29 ± 1.06ml/min/g at nitro stress, $p < 0.05$ both). Wall thickening at rest was higher in TMLR regions than in control regions of the same heart. (57 ± 7 vs $37\pm6\%$, $p<0.05$).

	Control	TMR
Delta EDV (μl)	24.6±16.7	81.7±15.7*
Delta LV mass (mg)	54.5±19.2	124.1±30.7*
EF at 12 weeks (%)	40±2	38±2
CI at 12 weeks (ml/kg/min)	232.2±12.8	242.4±12.8
EF at 12 weeks stress (%)	43±5	54±5*

Mean±SEM. *$p < 0.05$ vs control, delta: difference 8 vs 12 weeks after MI. EDV: end-diastolic volume, LV : left ventricle, EF: ejection fraction, CI: cardiac index. MI-size 27±2% both groups.

Using high resolution perfusion NMR, improvement of perfusion by TMLR was visualized. Due to the retrograde perfusion setting of the isolated heart this improvement cannot be caused by flow from inside the LV cavity via open channels. Translation of the results into the patients situation is not straight forward, however, some conclusions can be made. One explanation for the discrepancy of improved angina in patients after TMLR, but the failure of major studies to show improved perfusion may be insufficient spatial resolution of the applied imaging techniques. Addititonally, patients with impaired microcirculation may be successfully treated with TMLR. In relation to the left ventricular size in the rat the diameter of the laser fiber was rather large, however, the finding of enhanced LV remodeling should lead to additonal caution for the application of TMLR in the situation of post MI remodeling.

4.2 Influence of Testosterone on Cardiac Remodeling after Myocardial Infarction in Rats

Several facts suggest, that left ventricular remodeling after myocardial infarction may be influenced by androgen levels [6-8]. There is evidence of testosterone receptors in the heart. Further, it has been shown that testosterone use in bodybilders leads to increased left ventricular mass and rhythm abnormalities. Additionally, there is a large body of evidence for gender differences in pathophysiological processes in cardiovascular disease, for instance a lower incidence of myocardial infarction in premenopausal women. Aim of the study was to assess the influence of androgen levels on left ventricular remodeling after myocardial infarction (MI) in the intact rat. Wistar rats were assigned to 3 groups: surgical removal of testes 2 weeks prior to MI (ORX), Placebo (PL) and Testosterone-undekanoat-Injection (TUD, 500mg intramuscular 2 weeks prior to and 2 weeks after MI). NMR-measurements were done 2 and 8 weeks after left coronary artery ligation. Left ventricular (LV) mass and volumes, cardiac output (CO), ejection fraction (EF), wall thickness (WT) and – thickening (SWT) were determined. In addition, a transversal gradient echo of the paravertebral region was acquired to evaluate the growth of sceletal muscle.

	ORX (n=13)	Placebo (n=13)	TUD (n=9)
MI size 2 weeks (%)	36.4±2.0	38.8±2.9	37.7±1.8
Δ EDV (μl)	+276.0±33.2	+263.9±41.2	+245.6±51.2
Δ LV mass (mg)	+82.7±29	+170.7±43.6	+274.2±65.9*
CO 8 weeks (ml/min)	104.8±7.2	103.5±10.3	102.0±4.7
EF 8 weeks (%)	36±3	33±4	35±2
SWT 8 weeks (%)	66±7	34±3*	30±4*
PM (mm^2)	145.3±4.4	168.0±4.5*	187.8±5.3*†

Mean±SEM. * $p < 0.05$ vs.ORX, † 4 $p < 0.05$ vs. Placebo. Δ: difference from 2 to 8 weeks after MI. EDV: end-diastolic volume, PM: area of parevertebral sceletal muscle.

Dilation and global LV function after MI was not changed by manipulation of androgen levels, but hypertrophy was. Regional wall thickening of the remote region was preserved in ORX. In ORX growth of sceletal muscle was impaired and accelerated in TUD.

4.3 Impact of Cerivastatin on Cardiac Remodeling after Myocardial Infarction

Statin therapy has been shown to lower the incidence of myocardial infarction via positive effects in atherosclerosis [9]. Recently, it has been reported that statins have effects other than lipid lowering, and treatment after MI may be beneficial not only due to secondary prevention of reinfarction [10]. The influence of long-term cerivastatin therapy on left ventricular remodeling was assessed in rats with chronic myocardial infarction. In addition, the contribution of endogenous nitric oxide (NO) formation was assessed in animals treated with the NO synthase inhibitor L-NAME in combination with hydralazine (to avoid the increase in blood pressure induced by L-NAME). Using NMR it was possible to serially determine left ventricular mass as the most exact parameter of hypertrophy .

NMR-measurements were done 4 and 12 weeks after left coronary artery ligation. Rats were treated either with placebo, with cerivastatin (C, 0.6 mg/kg body weight) starting on the 7th postoperative day as dietary supplement, or cerivastatin plus L-NAME (76 mg/100 ml) and hydralazine (8 mg/100 ml) in drinking water (CLH)) daily for 12 weeks.

	Sham/ Placebo (n=8)	MI/ Placebo (n=8)	Cerivastatin (n=11)	CLH (n=11)
MI size 4 weeks (%)	0	31.5±2.7	31.9±1.4	31.9±2.8
Δ EDV (µl)	+26.8±20.4	+108.7±28.8*	+126.6±20.5*	+173.7±25.1*
Δ LV mass (mg)	+25.3±8.6	+235.3±33.7*	+59.8±20.5†	+239.5±16.0*‡
CO 12 weeks (ml/min)	73.0±3.6	76.1±2.9	95.8±4.8*†	69.3±2.8‡
EF 12 weeks (%)	70.1±2.0	36.2±3.1*	40.7±3.1*	33.0±2.6*‡
Δ EDWT (mm)	0.0±0.06	+0.5±0.06*	-0.08±0.06†	+0.4±0.06*‡
SWT 12 weeks (%)	80.9±6.9	32.5±4.4*	48.4±4.5†	29±2*‡

Mean±SEM. * p < 0.01 vs. Sham/Placebo, † p < 0.01 vs. MI/Placebo, ‡ p < 0.01 vs. Cerivastatin. Δ: difference from 4 to 12 weeks after MI. EDV: end-diastolic volume.

Administration of Cerivastatin attenuated left ventricular hypertrophy after MI. Dilation was not changed. Cardiac output and wall thickening were higher in Cerivastatin treated rats. The positive effects of Cerivastatin were completely abolished by NO synthase-inhibition.

4 Discussion

In the validation study NMR was shown to correlate closely to invasive or ex vivo techniques that are typically used in the rat model of myocardial infarction. With the advantage of its non-invasive character, NMR allows for serial investigations of the same animal. Hence, changes due to therapy or interventions can be monitored closely and more exact. Small differences can be detected, and the number of animals to be sacrified for research purposes can be reduced.

In conclusion we could show that Cine-MRI is a valuable diagnostic tool applicable to the rat model of myocardial infarction, which is in good agreement with existing analytical methods. It allows for reliable and reproducible assessment of cardiac morphology and function making it the method of choice for volumetric quantification. In contrast to echocardiography NMR-volumetry works without geometrical assumptions and therefore offers a high degree of accuracy in measurements of cardiac output and LV volumes; this is especially of importance in hearts deformed by asymmetric dilation after MI. NMR can be applied to assess the effects of therapeutical or other agents on infarct size, cardiac geometry and function with high precision. Thus NMR bears a great potential to substantially contribute to the understanding of the underlying pathomechanisms in the development of chronic heart failure and can help to evaluate new therapy options.

References

1. Pfeffer JM, Pfeffer MA, Braunwald E. Influence of chronic captopril therapy on the infarcted left ventricle of the rat. Circ Res 1985;57:84-95.
2. Pfeffer MA, Pfeffer JM, Fishbein MC, Fletcher J, Spadaro J, Kloner RA, Braunwald E. Myocardial infarct size and ventricular function in rats. Circ Res 1979;44:503-512.
3. Pfeffer MA, Frohlich ED. Electromagnetic flowmetry in anesthetized rats. J Appl Physiol 1972;33:137-140. 3. Fletcher PJ, Pfeffer MJ, Pfeffer MA, Braunwald E. Left ventricular diastolic pressure-volume relations in rats with healed myocardial infarction. Circ Res 1981;49:618-626.
4. Haase A, Frahm J, Matthaei M, Hänicke W, Merboldt KD. FLASH imaging: rapid NMR imaging using low flip angle pulses. J Magn Reson 1986;67:258-266.
5. Bauer WR, Hiller KH, Galuppo P, Neubauer S, Kopke J, Haase A, Waller C, Ertl G. Fast high resolution magnetic resonance imaging demonstrates fractality of myocardial perfusion in microscopic dimensions. Circ Res. 2001;88(3):340-346.
6. Scheuer J, Malhotra A, Schaible TF, Capasso J. Effects of gonadectomy and hormonal replacement on rat hearts. Circ Res 1987;61:12-19.
7. Webb CM, McNeill JG, Hayward CS, de Zeigler D, Collins P. Effects of Testosterone on coronary vasomotor regulation in men with coronary heart disease. Circulation 1999;100:1690-1696.
8. Marsh JD, Lehmann MH, Ritchie RH, Gwathmey JK, Green GE, Schiebinger RJ. Androgen receptors mediate hypertrophy in cardiac myocytes. Circulation 1998;98:256-261.
9. Scandinavian Simvastatin Study Group. Randomized trial of cholesterol lowering in 4444 patients with coronary artery disease: The Scandinavian Simvastatin Survival Study. Lancet 1994;344:1383-1389.
10. Wilson SH, Simari RD, Best PJ, Peterson DE, Lerman LO, Aviram M, Nath KA, Holmes DR Jr, Lerman A. Simvastatin preserves endothelial function in hypercholesterolemia in the absence of lipid lowering. Arterioscler Thromb Vasc Biol 2001;21(1):122-128.

Dempster Shafer Approach for High Level Data Fusion Applied to the Assessment of Myocardial Viability

Chantal Muller, Michèle Rombaut, and Marc Janier

CREATIS UMR CNRS 5515
69621 Villeurbanne France,
{rombaut, muller}@creatis.insa-lyon.fr

Abstract. A modular data fusion system based on the Dempster-Shafer framework is presented. This system allows the building of any architecture of fusion by chaining elementary modules. Two types of modules are used, the numerical to symbolic conversion modules and the combination modules using logical rules of combination. The uncertainty is modeled by a basic belief assignment or the plausibility of each hypothesis. We applied our system to assess the Left Ventricular (LV) myocardial viability. The parameters taken into account are the LV contractile function extracted from tagged Magnetic Resonance Images (MRI) and the glucose metabolism rate obtained by Positron Emission Tomography (PET) imaging. The variables of interest are defined by the medical experts. The results are displayed on polar maps to give a geometrical information of the potential lesions.

1 The Modular Fusion System

Medical diagnosis such as myocardial viability results from the integration of many complex phenomena which can not be precisely described by the specialists. Moreover, medical knowledge continuously evolves and research results lead to take into account new parameters. Our modular fusion system is designed to be adaptive to this uncertainty and this evolution. It allows medical specialists to experiment and analyze new architecture of fusion by combining the parameters according to their choice. This system enables to build any architecture of fusion. An architecture of fusion defines the scheme of data processing. It consists of a set of chained modules, classified in two types : the numerical to symbolic conversion modules (named Num2Sym modules) and the combination modules. The first modules are used for symbolic interpretation of the numerical reports from the sensors. The second ones perform the combination of these symbolic data in order to get synthetical information useful for diagnosis.

Running the algorithms of these modules needs a priori knowledge which is : (a) in case of Num2Sym modules, the model of the symbols defined on the reference of the numerical reports, (b) in case of combination modules, the logical rules of combination which define the symbolic values of the output from the

T. Katila et al. (Eds.): FIMH 2001, LNCS 2230, pp. 104–112, 2001.

symbolic values of the inputs. In this work, a priori knowledge will be provided by medical experts. In figure 1, an example of a simple architecture of fusion is presented for two inputs parameters X and Y. The numerical inputs are represented in italic in grey ellipsoids. These inputs are converted to symbolic data by Num2Sym modules, giving the symbolic data in white ellipsoids. These data are finally fused to get the output parameter Z.

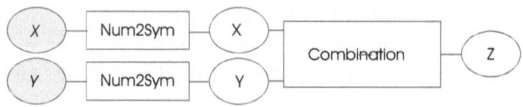

Fig. 1. Simple architecture of fusion

2   Dempster Shafer Framework

Our system is based on the Dempster-Shafer framework [1,2,3], well-adapted to model the uncertainty of the data and the rules of decision.

Model of the numerical to symbolic conversion. Each numerical parameter X taking x value in the interval I_X is linked to a set of hypothesis $\Omega_X = \{H_X^i / i = 1, N\}$, N the number of hypothesis. It is proposed to define a trapezoïdal function $f_{H_X^i}$ assigned to each hypothesis H_X^i on the interval I_X, but also to each proposition A_X^i stemmed from the logical union of several hypothesis. In fact, the medical expert always defines ordered hypothesis on the interval I_X with inaccurate thresholds, so we propose to model the doubt between to consecutive hypothesis by a composed hypothesis or proposition such as $(H_X^i \cup H_X^{i+1})$ where $\cup$ corresponds to the union of the two hypothesis, such as represented Figure 2. The function m_x, called basic belief assignment, models the confidence that a numerical value $x \in I_X$ belongs to the different propositions A_X^i defined by subsets of Ω_X. The definition of m_x is :

$$m_x : 2^{\Omega_X} \rightarrow [0,1]$$
$$A_X^i \mapsto m_x(A_X^i) = f_{A_X^i}(x) \tag{1}$$

We deliberately choose a simple model, because it is well-adapted to translate the medical expertise. In our application, propositions given by experts are ordered on the numerical space of definition I_X, only the thresholds between two consecutive propositions are not accurate.

Model of combination rules. The combination of two symbolic variables gives a third symbolic variable that must be interpreted by the medical experts.

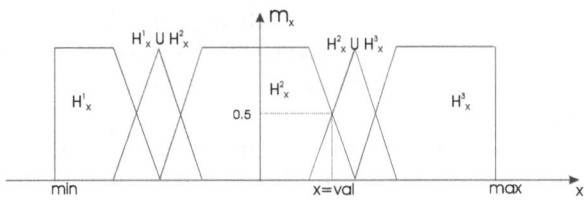

Fig. 2. Model of the numerical - symbolic transformation

The basic combination rules are extensively described by a decision table from the a priori knowledge of the clinical experts. Let $\Omega_X = \{H_X^1, H_X^2, H_X^3\}$, $\Omega_Y = \{H_Y^1, H_Y^2, H_Y^3\}$ and $\Omega_Z = \{H_Z^1, H_Z^2, H_Z^3\}$ be the sets of hypothesis respectively related to the symbolic variables X, Y and Z. Table 1 exhibits an example of rules determining the output variable Z from the combination of X and Y.

Table 1. Basic rules of combination defined from X and Y for the determination of Z

		X hypothesis		
	Z	H_X^1	H_X^2	H_X^3
Y	H_Y^1	H_Z^1	H_Z^1	H_Z^1
hypothesis	H_Y^2	H_Z^2	H_Z^3	H_Z^1
	H_Y^3	H_Z^2	H_Z^2	H_Z^2

The combination is based on the unnormalised form of the Dempster's conjunctive rule. This rule allows the combination of two distributions defined on the same space of discernment. Nevertheless, it is possible to extend this rule, if a logical table of combination such as Table 1 is known. An illustration is given with the following simple example. Let

$$m_x : 2^{\Omega_X} \to [0,1]$$
$$\Omega_X = \{H_X^1, H_X^2\} \tag{2}$$

$$m_y : 2^{\Omega_Y} \to [0,1]$$
$$\Omega_Y = \{H_Y^1, H_Y^2\} \tag{3}$$

be the basic believe assignments of the numerical parameters X and Y. m_x and m_y can be redefined by m_x' and m_y' on the discernment space

$$\Omega_X \otimes \Omega_Y = \{(H_X^1 \cap H_Y^1), (H_X^1 \cap H_Y^2), (H_X^2 \cap H_Y^1), (H_X^2 \cap H_Y^2)\}$$

$$m_x(H_X^i) = m_x'((H_X^i \cap H_Y^1) \cup (H_X^i \cap H_Y^2))$$
$$= m_x'(H_X^i \cap (H_Y^1 \cup H_Y^2))$$
$$m_x(H_X^1 \cup H_X^2) = m_x'((H_X^1 \cap H_Y^1) \cup (H_X^1 \cap H_Y^2) \cup (H_X^2 \cap H_Y^1) \cup (H_X^2 \cap H_Y^2))$$
$$= m_x'((H_X^1 \cup H_X^2) \cap (H_Y^1 \cup H_Y^2))$$

The same extension can be made with m_y to m'_y. Thus, m'_x and m'_y are defined on the same space of discernment. The Dempster's combination rule can be used given $m'_Z = m'_x \oplus m'_y$, where m'_Z is defined on $\Omega_X \otimes \Omega_Y$ for the two measures x and y.

We can notice that this extension increases the dimension of the space of discernment. $Dim(\Omega_X) = 2$ and $Dim(\Omega_Y) = 2$, so $Dim(\Omega_X \otimes \Omega_Y) = 4$. In many cases, the expert gives an interpretation of the resulting hypothesis, defining the hypothesis of the result variable Z. For instance,

$$
\begin{aligned}
(H_X^1 \cap H_Y^1) &= H_Z^1 \\
(H_X^1 \cap H_Y^2) &= H_Z^2 \\
(H_X^2 \cap H_Y^1) &= H_Z^2 \\
(H_X^2 \cap H_Y^2) &= H_Z^3
\end{aligned}
\tag{4}
$$

This interpretation can be described by a logical array as shown in Table2. The transformation of m'_Z defined on $\Omega_X \otimes \Omega_Y$, to m_Z defined on Ω_Z is made by using equations (4).

Table 2. Interpretation of the resulting hypothesis

	$\mathbf{Z}$	H_X^1	H_X^2
Y	H_Y^1	H_Z^1	H_Z^2
$hypothesis$	H_Y^2	H_Z^2	H_Z^3

Xhypothesis

Practically, it is sufficient to extend the Table 2 from Ω to 2^Ω to get the new Table 3 that represents the Tab function, and to transform the Dempster's rule to:

$$
m_Z(A) = \sum_{A=Tab(B,C)} m_x(B).m_y(C)
$$

Table 3. Extension of the resulting hypothesis

Xhypothesis

	$\mathbf{Z}$	H_X^1	H_X^2	$H_X^1 \cup H_X^2$
Y	H_Y^1	H_Z^1	H_Z^2	$H_Z^1 \cup H_Z^2$
$hypothesis$	H_Y^2	H_Z^2	H_Z^3	$H_Z^2 \cup H_Z^3$
	$H_Y^1 \cup H_Y^2$	$H_Z^1 \cup H_Z^2$	$H_Z^2 \cup H_Z^3$	$H_Z^1 \cup H_Z^2 \cup H_Z^3$

Reports processing. Both models developed in the previous section are completely independent of the reports of a particular patient. They just model the knowledge of the medical experts. The reports processing uses the previous models. Given a numerical value x of the variable X, a basic belief assignment m_x is computed from the model of conversion previously defined in the module Num2Sym associated to this variable. The combination step needs the definition of a combination table. The belief assignment m_Z of the output variable Z is computed from the Dempster's conjunctive rule in unnormalized form.

3   Application to the Diagnosis of Myocardial Viability

Myocardial viability. Myocardial viability assessment is an important field of research in cardiac diseases. Viable tissue is under-perfused tissue that can recover after blood flow reestablishment. The quantification of the viable tissue is of major importance in medical diagnosis since it helps to decide whether or not a patient will benefit from a revascularisation procedure [4]. In order to make an automatic accurate viability analysis, complementary diagnosis parameters have to be integrated in to the system. It has been shown that the combination of the glucose metabolism and the LV contractile function gives a good assessment of the viability [5,6]. Contractile function analysis is obtained from tagged Magnetic Resonance Imaging (MRI). Glucose metabolism rate is provided by a Positron Emission Tomography (PET) scanner.

Input parameters. MR images of the heart are acquired using a Siemens Vision 1.5T scanner with 35ms temporal resolution (8mm slice thickness, 45 and 135 degree tag orientations, FOV 280mm). The investigation of LV function in tagged MR images is performed with a cardiac analysis package (*FindTags*, John Hokkins University, Baltimore). Two parameters are considered for the assessment of the LV contractile function: the Maximum circumferential Shortening (MS) of deformation tensor and the Angle (A) formed by displacement vector versus the circumferential direction. Both parameters are computed on rest images (MSr, Ar) and stress images (MSs, As) at end diastole. PET volume (64 slices) are acquired on a HR+ tomograph (Siemens Erlangen) in 3D mode with intrinsic resolution of (4mm x 4mm x 4mm). One hour after initiation of euglycemic hyperinsulinemic clamp infusion, 3 to 4 mCi of 18FDG are injected as a slow bolus. The studied volume is taken 45 min after this infusion with 15mn acquisition time. The uptake rate (FDG) (glucose metabolism parameter) of any myocardial region is obtained by counting procedure. A major problem in fusion system is data registration. In our application, this step is previously performed using a semi-automatic software (*Cardiofuz*, CREATIS, Lyon). Our modular fusion system will use five input parameters: MSr, Ar, MSs, As and FDG. The format of these data will be uniformed and fits well to a standard polar map display.

Architecture of the fusion system. Such as presented Figure 3, the numerical inputs of MSr, Ar, MSs, As and FDG are converted into symbolic data by Num2Sym modules, giving the symbolic data in white ellipsoids. These data are finally fused two by two until to get the needed results which is the viability ($Viab$). Intermediate variables are derived from the initial ones: the contractile function at rest (CRr), the contractile function under stress (CFs), the inotropic function based on CFr and CFs comparison (IF) and the viability $Viab$.

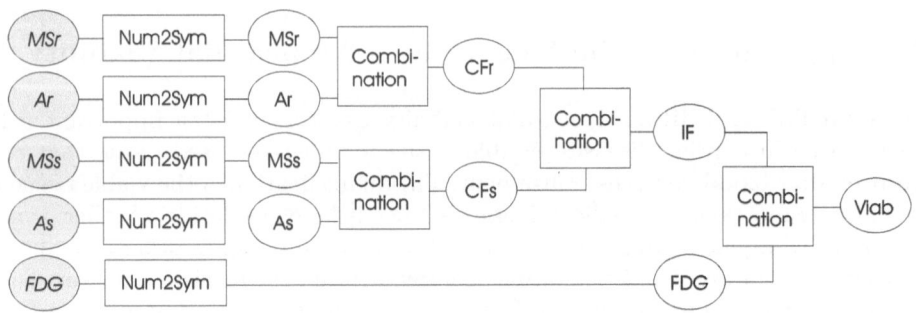

Fig. 3. Architecture of fusion

Models of the numerical to symbolic conversion. Num2Sym modules are configured in order to make the conversion of the numerical values of MSs, MSr, Ar, As and FDG into symbolic data. The hypothesis and the basic belief assignments of each numerical variables are defined with medical experts. The symbolic variables obtained from the numerical variables are described in Table 4. For instance, the MSs variable is associated by the medical expert to three hypothesis, then $\Omega_{MSs} = \{N, Z, P\}$. Each trapezoidal function f_N, f_Z, f_P and of course $f_{N\cup Z}$, $f_{Z\cup P}$ is also defined by the expert. These definitions allow the system to make the numerical/symbolic conversion as presented section 2.

Table 4. Single hypothesis of the symbolic input variables

MSs		As		MSr		Ar		FDG	
N	Negative	N	Negative	S	Small	S	Small	S	Small
Z	Zero	Z	Zero	L	Large	L	Large	M	Medium
P	Positive	P	Positive					L	Large

Models of combination. Table 5 describes the symbolic variables CFr, CFs, IF and $Viab$ derived from the symbolic input variables MSr, MSs, Ar, As and FDG. The basic rules of combination are represented by logical arrays. Table 6 summarizes these combination rules for all symbolic output variables used in the architecture of fusion.

Table 5. Single hypothesis of the symbolic output variables

CFs		CFr		IF	
Lr	Lower	ADK	Akinetic	ANI	Akinetic at rest and no improvement
Eq	Equal	HK	Hypokinetic	HNI	Hypokinetic at rest and no improvement
Hr	Higher	NL	Normal	FI	Function improvement
				I	Ischemic
				R	Remote

Viab			
Er	Error : FDG /IF Mismatch	V	Viable
NE	Necrosis	I	Ischemic
Md	Maimed	R	Remote
MV	Metabolic Viable		

Table 6. Basic rules of combination used by the architecture of fusion

MSr

	CFr	S	L
Ar S		HK	NL
L		ADK	ADK

MSs

	CFs	N	Z	P
As N		Hr	Hr	Hr
Z		Lr	Eq	Hr
P		Lr	Lr	Lr

CFr

	IF	ADK	HK	NL
CFs Lr		ANI	HNI	I
Eq		ANI	HNI	R
Hr		FI	FI	R

IF

	Viab	ANI	HNI	FI	I	R
FDG S		Ne	Md	Er	Er	Er
M		Md	Md	V	I	R
L		MV	MV	V	I	R

For instance, the belief basic assignment of the MSs and Ar variables are combined using the method presented in section 2 to give belief basic assignment of CFs variable. The space of discernment of CFs is then $\Omega_{CFs} = \{Lr, Eq, Hr\}$.

Results. The medical experts need to know where a risk may occur, so we chose to show them the plausibility of each hypothesis of the final variable which is the viability. The plausibilities of each hypothesis presented in Table 5 are computed. The results obtained from the data of a particular patient are displayed on polar maps Figure 4.

4   Conclusion

A modular data fusion system was developed with Dempster-Shafer framework. It is based on modules of two types: the Num2Sym modules parameterized by

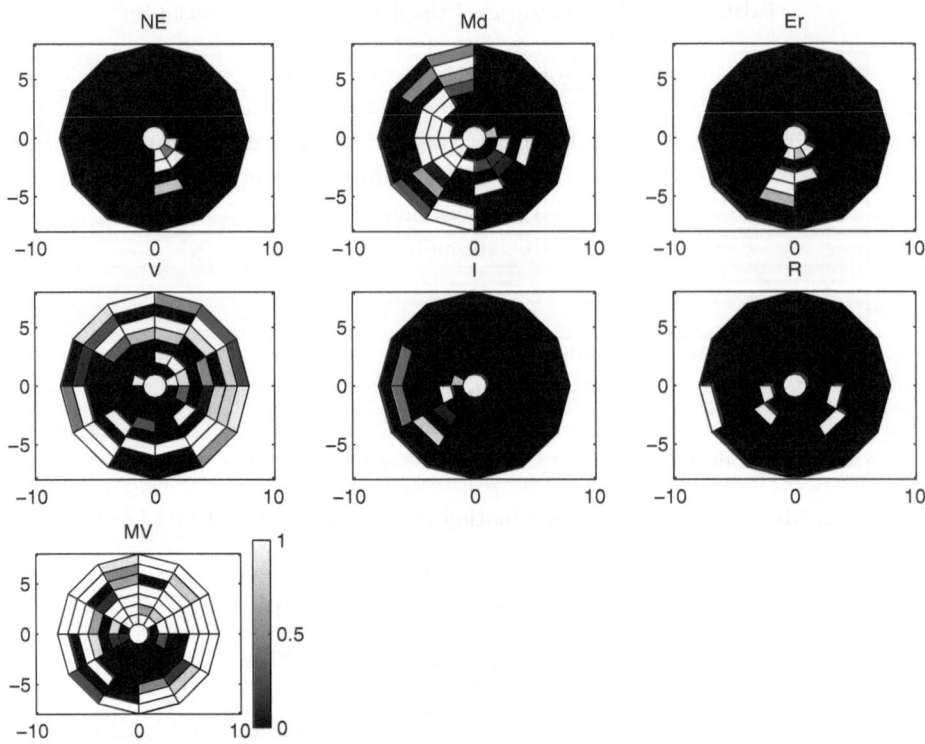

Fig. 4. The polar maps of the plausibility for the different hypothesis of the viability

the thresholds and the frame of the conversion and the Combination modules easily definable to fit to the specialists knowledge. Thus, any architecture of fusion may be built from these modules.

This system is a sort of rules base system, but taking into account the uncertainty on the data, modeled by a basic belief assignment. Similar results might be obtained with a fuzzy rule base system. The choice of the Dempster Shafer theory has been approved by the medical expert because of its ability to model the doubt.

An architecture of fusion has been implemented to assess the myocardial viability. The diagnosis results from the processing of five input parameters CFr, CFs, Ar, As and FDG associated to LV contractile function and the glucose metabolism. It is displayed on polar maps, using the mass of evidence or the plausibility of each hypothesis. In a future work, we will assess the accuracy of the diagnosis by comparing our results to the real measurements performed on 30 patients before and after a revascularisation procedure.

References

1. G. Schafer. *A mathematical theory of evidence*, volume 2702. Princetown University Press, 1976.
2. A. Dempster. A generalization of bayesian inference. *Journal of the Royal Statistical Society*, **30**:205–247, 1968.
3. P. Smets. What is dempster-Shafer's model? Technical Report TR/IRIDIA/Sl-20, IRIDIA-Universiti, Libre de Bruxelles, 50 Av F. Roosevelt. CP194/6. B-1050 Bruxelles, 1991.
4. Behloul F., M.Janier, P.Croisille, C. Poirier, A. Boudraa, R.Unterreiner, J.C. Mason, and D. Revel. Automatic assessment of myocardial viability based on pet-mri data fusion. *In Proceeding of the 20th Annual International Conference of the IEEE Engineering in Medicine and Biology Society*, pages 492–495, 1998.
5. Behloul F., M.Janier, P.Croisille, C. Poirier, A. Boudraa, R.Unterreiner, J.C. Mason, and D. Revel. Mri-pet data fusion using soft computing for the automatic assessment of myocardial viability. *Computers in cardiology*, 25, 1998.
6. D.L. Kraitchman, A.A. Young, D.C. Bloomgarden, Z.A. Fayad, L. Dougherty, V.A. Ferrari, R.C. Boston, and L. Axel. Integrated mri assessment of regional function and perfusion in canine myocardial infarction. *Magnetic Resonance in Medicine*, **40**(2):311–326, August 1998.

Experimental and Computational Modeling of Cardiac Electromechanical Coupling

Andrew D. McCulloch, Derrick Sung, Mary Ellen Thomas, and
Anushka Michailova

Department of Bioengineering, The Whitaker Institute for Biomedical Engineering
University of California San Diego
La Jolla, California

1 Introduction

Perturbations in ventricular mechanical loading can be arrhythmogenic and have been associated with sudden cardiac death in patients suffering from congestive heart failure, dilated cardiomyopathy, or ventricular volume overload (1-3). Stretch-induced changes in action potential propagation or repolarization could provide a mechanism for mechanically induced arrhythmias. However, there is a paucity of information regarding the effects of altered load on conduction velocity. The few existing reports present an unclear picture; some of the discrepancies may be due to the varying techniques used.

Stretch activated channels (SACs) have been identified as a potential cellular mechanism for mechanoelectric feedback (4). Mechano-sensitive ion channels have been identified in the ventricular myocardium of several species, both non-specific cation or K^+ specific channels (5-7). The aminoglycoside antibiotic streptomycin has been reported to block stretch activated channels (8).

Past studies of cardiac mechanoelectric feedback have all used contact electrodes to measure the electrical activity of the heart. The required physical contact between the measuring device and the myocardium leaves the measurements open to the possibility of mechanically induced electrical artifact (9). Optical mapping provides a non-contact means of measuring cardiac electrical activity through the use of a voltage-sensitive fluorescent dye. The spatial resolution from this technique is higher than that of conventional electrode arrays and is thus particularly desirable for conduction velocity measurements. In the present study, we employed optical mapping to investigate the effects of increased left ventricular loading on apparent epicardial conduction velocity and action potential duration. Streptomycin was used to assess if any of the observed electrophysiological changes might be governed by stretch activated channels. A preliminary report of this study has appeared in the proceedings of the 2001 ASME Summer Bioengineering meeting (10).

Computational models are also valuable tools for investigating cardiac electromechanical interactions. By adding stretch activated currents to ionic models of the cardiac myocyte action potential, the integrated effects on stretch on cardiac electrophysiology can be investigated (11). These models can then be integrated into three-dimensional continuum analyses of ventricular mechanics and action potential propagation. This work has all been previously reported in full or preliminary reports (10, 12-17).

T. Katila et al. (Eds.): FIMH 2001, LNCS 2230, pp. 113-119, 2001.
© Springer-Verlag Berlin Heidelberg 2001

2 Experimental Methods

Experiments were conducted in isolated Langendorff-perfused rabbit hearts. A balloon in the left ventricle was connected to a fluid-filled pressure transducer and a volume infusion pump. Following aortic cannulation, hearts were perfused with Tyrode's solution and allowed to actively contract. The initial volume in the balloon was adjusted to achieve an end diastolic pressure (EDP) of ≈0 mmHg. Hearts were perfused with a bolus of the voltage-sensitive dye, DI-4-ANEPPS and loaded from 0-30 mm Hg left ventricular pressure at a constant rate. Just prior to the acquisition of optical measurements, the electromechanical uncoupler 2,3 butanedione monoxime (BDM, 12.5 mM) was also added to the perfusate to prevent motion artifact. The heart was paced at a cycle length of 300 msec from the left ventricular epicardium near the apex. The loading protocol was repeated after the perfusate was switched to one containing 200•M streptomycin.

The hardware configuration for optical mapping has been described previously (18). Fluorescence images of the LV free wall (lateral view) were captured with a digital CCD camera (Dalsa, Waterloo, Ontario) at a speed of 399 frames per second and a resolution of 128×128 pixels. The image processing and analysis of the optical data has been detailed elsewhere (18, 19). After the signals were filtered, activation times were identified as the time at the maximum first derivative (dF/dt)max of the optical action potential upstroke. Time of repolarization was computed by determining the time at which the optical action potential had recovered 20% and 80% from its peak. The difference between the repolarization and activation times was taken to be the action potential duration (APD).

The epicardial geometry of each heart was reconstructed from orthogonal biplane images of the lateral and posterior views, and a finite-element surface was then fitted to the boundary data yielding a three-dimensional model of the epicardium. The activation times, maximum derivatives of the upstroke, and action potential duration times were then mapped on to the surface of the finite element model and fit by linear least squares. This allowed the electrophysiological variables to be expressed as functions of the three-dimensional coordinates of the epicardial geometry.

3 Results

Epicardial activation times were reversibly prolonged during loading (Fig. 1). Total mean apparent conduction velocity averaged over all distances decreased from about 400 mm/sec in the unloaded pre-control state to less than 300 mm/sec in the loaded state ($p < 0.05$). By ANOVA, the interaction effect between load state and distance from pacing site was not significant suggesting that the decrease in conduction velocity was not changed at the different locations on the surface of the heart. There was no significant change in apparent conduction velocity between the two unloaded states. (dF/dt)max of the optical action potential upstroke decreased about 5%, but a decrease of this amount or greater would be expected simply as a result of slowed conduction, so decreased membrane excitability is unlikely to explain the observed stretch-dependent slowing. Adding streptomycin to the perfusate did not change the overall conduction velocities or the response of apparent conduction velocity to load, suggesting that SACs may not play a primary role in this effect. There was no significant difference in the relative decrease in apparent conduction velocity with respect to distance from the pacing site, suggesting that the effect may be present transmurally throughout the myocardium.

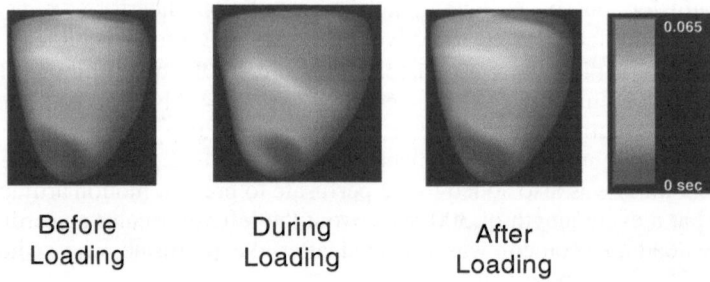

Before
Loading

During
Loading

After
Loading

Fig. 1. Epicardial activation times in unloaded (left and right) and loaded (center) rabbit left ventricle. From (12)

Total mean APD_{20} increased a mean of 13 msec when load was applied ($p < 0.05$) and recovered following removal of the load. Mean APD_{80} increased by 28 msec following the application of ventricular load ($p < 0.0001$) but only recovered partially by 1 min after removal of the load. Streptomycin. Streptomycin did not have a significant effect on APD and did not affect the response of APD_{20} or APD_{80} to changes in ventricular loading states.

4   Model Analysis

We investigated the possibility that altered intracellular calcium cycling via length-dependent activation may contribute to the increase in APD with stretch. Using a modification by Michailova and McCulloch (13) (Fig. 2) of the canine ionic model by Winslow et al (20), we simulated the effects of stretch by increasing the on-rate for calcium binding to troponin and studied the influence on action potential duration. This preliminary analysis showed that under some circumstances the resulting decrease in free myoplasmic calcium during systole was able to prolong relaxation somewhat (Fig. 3).

Mechanoelectric feedback has been described in isolated cells and intact ventricular myocardium, but the mechanical stimulus that governs mechanosensitive channel activity in intact tissue is unknown. To investigate the effects of stretch-activated currents on regional action potential propagation in three-dimensions, we developed a finite element model of electromechanics in the rabbit heart. An anatomically detailed model of rabbit right and left ventricular geometry and fiber architecture was developed (15) and used to model regional mechanics during filling (16). See Fig. 4. The resulting strain field was then used as a stimulus for regional stretch-activated current (17). A stretch-dependent current was added in parallel to the ionic currents in the Beeler-Reuter ventricular action potential model (Fig. 5). Electrical propagation was simulated using the collocation-Galerkin finite element method. We investigated different mechanical coupling parameters to simulate stretch-dependent conductance modulated by either fiber strain, cross-fiber strain, or a

116   A.D. McCulloch et al.

combination of the two. In response to pressure loading, the conductance model governed by fiber strain alone reproduced the epicardial decrease in action potential amplitude as observed in experimental preparations of the passively loaded rabbit heart (21). The model governed by only cross-fiber strain reproduced the transmural gradient in action potential amplitude as observed in isolated heart experiments, but failed to predict a sufficient decrease in amplitude at the epicardium. Only the model governed by both fiber and cross-fiber strain reproduced the epicardial and transmural changes in action potential amplitude similar to experimental observations (21). In addition, dispersion of action potential duration nearly doubled with the same model. These results suggest that changes in action potential characteristics may be due not only to length changes along the long axis direction of the myofiber, but also due to deformation in the plane transverse to the fiber axis. The model provides a framework for investigating how cellular biophysics affect the function of the intact ventricles.

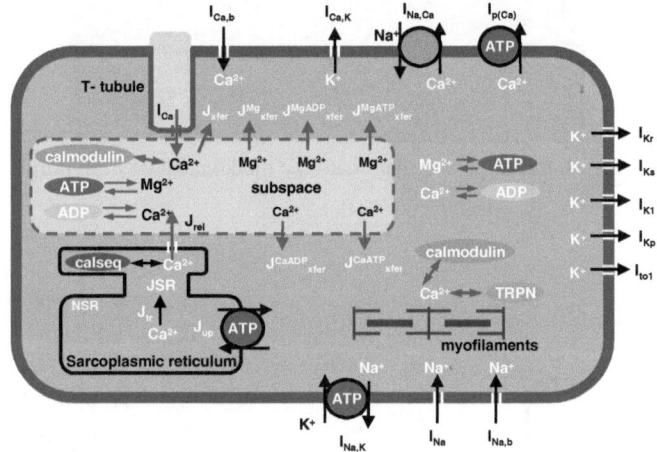

Fig. 2. Myocyte ionic model, adapted from (13)

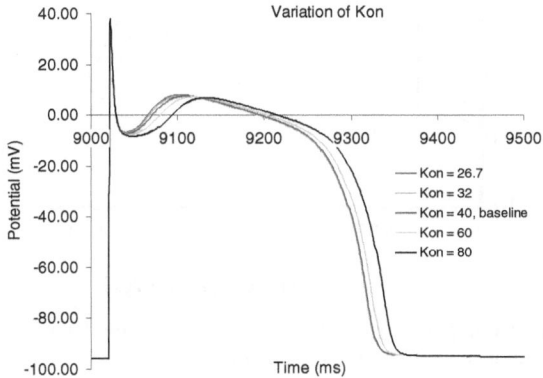

Fig. 3. Increasing troponin affinity for calcium prolonged the action potential in a preliminary model. Adapted from (12)

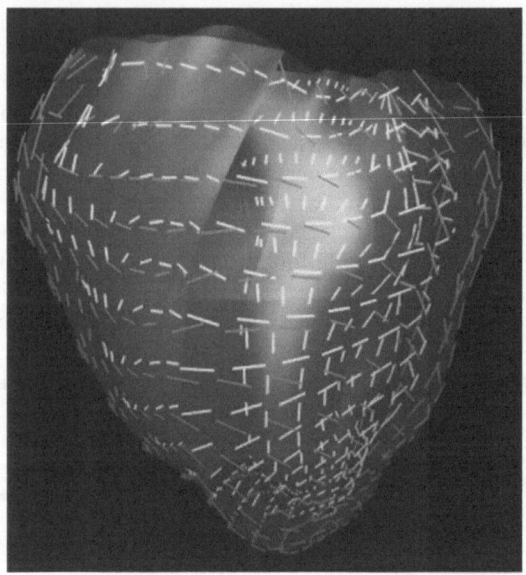

Fig. 4. Rabbit ventricular anatomic model adapted from (15)

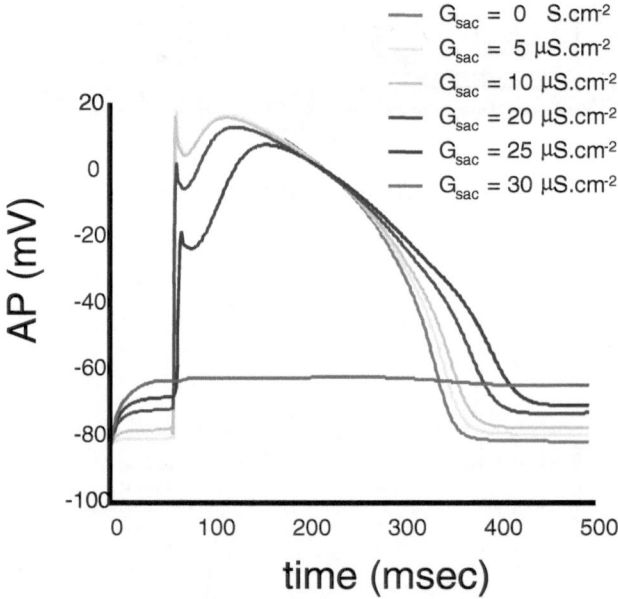

Fig. 5. Action potential computed from Beeler-Reuter ionic model with varying degrees of stretch-activated conductance, G_{sac}. Adapted from (11, 17).

5   Discussion

We have shown that acute loading of the left ventricle decreases apparent epicardial conduction velocity and increases action potential duration in the isolated rabbit heart and these responses do not appear to be mediated by a stretch-activated current. The decrease in conduction velocity could have potential arrhythmogenic consequences by decreasing the wavelength for reentry. In this way, mechanoelectric could contribute to arrhythmias associated with altered ventricular loading conditions. We also observed a prolongation of action potential duration with loading that was not blocked by streptomycin. A model analysis suggests that altered intracellular calcium cycling could be a contributing mechanism. Three-dimensional models provide a framework for integrating coupled cardiac functions across scales of organization from myocyte to whole organ.

Acknowledgements. This research was supported in part by NSF grant BES-9634974 and the National Biomedical Computation Resource, NIH P41 grant RR08605. Derrick Sung was supported by NIH training grant T32HL07444. Mary Ellen Thomas was an NSF scholar.

Our modeling software can be downloaded free from http://cmrg.ucsd.edu/

References

1. Dean JW, Lab MJ. Arrhythmia in heart failure: role of mechanically induced changes in electrophysiology. Lancet 1989;8650(1):1309-1312.
2. Huang SK, Messer JV, Denes P. Significance of ventricular tachycardia in idiopathic dilated cardiomyopathy: observations in 35 patients. Am J Cardiol 1983;51(3):507-512.
3. Reiter MJ. Effects of mechano-electrical feedback: potential arrhythmogenic influence in patients with congestive heart failure. Cardiovascular Research 1996;32(1):44-51.
4. Hu H, Sachs F. Stretch-activated ion channels in the heart. J Mol Cell Cardiol 1997;29(6):1511-23.
5. Ruknudin A, Sachs F, Bustamante JO. Stretch-activated ion channels in tissue-cultured chick heart. Am J Physiol 1993;264:H960-H972.
6. Craelius W, Chen V, el-Sherif N. Stretch activated ion channels in ventricular myocytes. Bioscience Reports 1988;8(5):407-14.
7. Sigurdson W, Morris C, Brezden B, Gardner D. Stretch activation of a K^+ channel in colluscan heart cells. Journal of Experimental Biology 1987;127:191-209.
8. Salmon AH, Mays JL, Dalton GR, Jones JV, Levi AJ. Effect of streptomycin on wall-stress-induced arrhythmias in the working rat heart. Cardiovasc Res 1997;34(3):493-503.
9. Lab MJ. Mechanoelectric feedback (transduction) in heart: concepts and implications. Cardiovasc Res 1996;32(1):3-14.
10. Sung D, Omens JH, McCulloch AD. Ventricular mechanoelectric feedback in the isolated rabbit heart. In: Kamm RD, Schmid-Schonbein GW, Ateshian GA, Hefzy MS, editors. Summer Bioengineering Conference; 2001; Snowbird, Utah; 2001. p. 683-684.
11. Rice JJ, Winslow RL, Dekanski J, McVeigh E. Model studies of the role of mechano-sensitive currents in the generation of cardiac arrhythmias. J Theor Biol 1998;190(4):295-312.

12. McCulloch A, Sung D, Thomas ME, Michailova A. Chapter 11: Computational and Experimental Modeling of Ventricular Electromechanical Interactions. In: Virag N, Blanc O, Kappenberger L, editors. Computer Simulation and Experimental Assessment of Cardiac Electrophysiology. Amonk, NY: Futura Publishing Company, Inc.; 2001. p. 89-94.
13. Michailova A, McCulloch AD. Modeling Ca^{2+} transients and Ca^{2+} and Mg^{2+} exchange with ATP and ADP during excitation-contraction coupling in ventricular myocytes. Biophys J 2001;81(2):614-629.
14. Sung D. Effects of Mechanical Load on Ventricular action Potential Propagation and Repolarization [Ph.D.]. La Jolla: University of California San Diego; 2001.
15. Vetter FJ, McCulloch AD. Three-dimensional analysis of regional cardiac function: a model of rabbit ventricular anatomy. Progress in Biophysics and Molecular Biology 1998;69(2-3):157-183.
16. Vetter FJ, McCulloch AD. Three-dimensional stress and strain in passive rabbit left ventricle: A model study. Ann Biomed Eng 2000;28:781-792.
17. Vetter FJ, McCulloch AD. Mechanoelectric feedback in a model of the passively inflated left ventricle. Ann Biomed Eng 2001;29:414-426 (and cover).
18. Sung D, Omens JH, McCulloch AD. Model-based analysis of optically mapped epicardial activation patterns and conduction velocity. Ann Biomed Eng 2000;28(9):1085-1092.
19. Sung D, Somayajula-Jagai J, Cosman P, McCulloch AD. Phase-shifting prior to spatial filtering enhances optical recordings of cardiac action potential propagation. Ann Biomed Eng (in press) 2001.
20. Winslow RL, Rice J, Jafri S, Marban E, O'Rourke B. Mechanisms of altered excitation-contraction coupling in canine tachycardia-induced heart failure, II: model studies. Circ Res 1999;84(5):571-86.
21. Zabel M, Koller BS, Sachs F, Franz MR. Stretch-induced voltage changes in the isolated beating heart: importance of the timing of stretch and implications for stretch-activated ion channels. Cardiovascular Research 1996;32(1):120-30.

Towards Model-Based Estimation of the Cardiac Electro-Mechanical Activity from ECG Signals and Ultrasound Images

N. Ayache[1], D. Chapelle[3], F. Clément[4], Y. Coudière[2], H. Delingette[1], J.A. Désidéri[2], M. Sermesant[*1], M. Sorine[4], and J.M. Urquiza[3]

[1] ÉPIDAURE Research Project, INRIA Sophia Antipolis,
2004 route des Lucioles, 06902 Sophia Antipolis, France
[2] SINUS Research Project, INRIA Sophia Antipolis
[3] MACS Research Project, INRIA Rocquencourt
[4] SOSSO Research Project, INRIA Rocquencourt

Abstract. We present a 3D numerical representation of the heart which couples the electrical and biomechanical models. To achieve this, the FitzHugh-Nagumo equations are solved along with a constitutive law based on the Hill-Maxwell rheological law. Ultimately, the parameters of this generic model will be adjusted by comparing the actual patient's ECG with computational results and the deformation of the biomechanical model with the geometric information extracted from the ultrasound images of the patient's heart.

1 Introduction

The objective of our multidisciplinary project ICEMA (standing for Images of the Cardiac Electro-Mechanical Activity, a collaborative research action between different INRIA projects) is to build a generic dynamic model of the beating heart and a procedure to automatically adjust the parameters to any specific patient. We plan to construct an identification procedure using 2 sets of relatively easy-to-access measurements on a patient: the ECG (Electrocardiogram), and a time sequence of volumetric ultrasound images. Once the generic model is adapted to a specific patient, it becomes possible to derive a set of quantitative and objective parameters useful in helping clinicians and physiologists to better understand the electro-mechanical coupling and diagnose pathological conditions. Significant results are expected in the following fields of cardiovascular pathology:

- assessment of the hæmodynamic repercussions of heart rate and electrical conduction disorders;
- assessment of the degree of heart failure (inefficiency of the cardiac pump induced by weakened cardiac contractility resulting in increased local wall thickness and decreased ejection fraction);

---

[*] Corresponding Author: Maxime.Sermesant@inria.fr

T. Katila et al. (Eds.): FIMH 2001, LNCS 2230, pp. 120–127, 2001.

– assessment of the electrical and mechanical repercussions of cardiac infarction (right ventricle infarction is believed to rather lead to electrical repercussions while left ventricle infarction is believed to lead to mechanical repercussions);

Our approach combines a 3D numerical model of the electric wave propagation with a 3D biomechanical model of the cardiac muscle. The 2 models are explicitly coupled in the simulation to generate a dynamic behaviour of the heart. The model for electric wave propagation is derived from FitzHugh-Nagumo equations, while the mechanical model is based on the classical Hill-Maxwell rheological law. These models are expected to reflect on a macroscopic scale the coupling present on the cellular scale. To provide a realistic motion of a standard beating heart, the highly anisotropic nature of the muscle fibres in standard anatomy are accounted for. The electric wave is propagated from the extremities of the Purkinje network.

Two error functions will serve to adjust the parameters of this generic model to a specific patient: the first will compare the actual patient's ECGs with a set of ECGs computed from the simulation. The second will compare the deformation of the biomechanical model with the motion extracted from the ultrasound images of the patient's heart. In addition, the ventricular blood pressure, when available, is readily introduced as a constraint for the deformation of the biomechanical model. Ultimately, a retro-action procedure will be used to update the parameters of the generic model from these error functions.

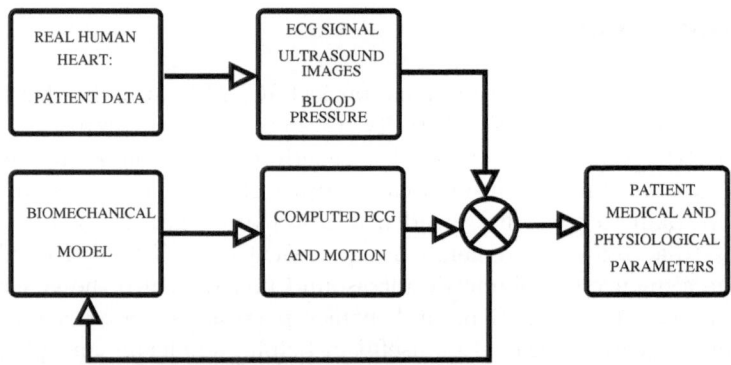

In this article, we develop the current stages of this on-going research. In section 2, we describe the construction of a finite element model incorporating standard anatomical knowledge. In sections 3 and 4 we respectively describe the electrical and mechanical models. Section 5 describes a preliminary approach to account for the geometric information provided by the ultrasound image sequence. Finally, section 6 discusses the possible refinements we plan to introduce in each of these models, and the directions towards the identification of the parameters of the global system.

2   Anatomical Model

2.1   Geometry and Muscle Fibres

Our geometric model consists of a mesh of the ventricular myocardium (including both right and left ventricles) and of the myocardium fibre directions. Indeed, the fibre architecture has a great influence on the motion and propagation of the electrical excitation. The model is based on data available from the Bioengineering Research Group of the University of Auckland, New Zealand [9]. These data have been obtained by the dissection of a dog's heart and are composed of a mesh with 256 nodes, 180 hexahedra, and fibre direction at each node.

Since these data are too coarse for 3D computations, new meshes have been generated using a procedure which consists in:

1. interpolating the surface of the mesh with a mesh of triangles;
2. remeshing the 3D volume with tetrahedra;
3. interpolating the fibre directions on the new mesh.

We obtained meshes with 623, 3763, and 9623 vertices.

2.2   Conduction Network and Electrical Onset

A complete three-dimensional model of the heart should include both the cardiac muscle and special conduction network (Purkinje fibres and His bundle branches) [2,13] and whose role is rendered through boundary conditions: the fibres of Purkinje are assumed to end up within the muscle in a region of the endocardium; a pulse-shaped boundary condition is applied on this hand-delimited region as a model of onset of the cardiac excitation.

3   Electrical Model

Each heart-beat cycle, a depolarisation wave is initiated (see above) and propagates along the myocardium during about 10% of the total cardiac cycle.

Among the various models for the electric wave propagation, the FitzHugh-Nagumo model is classical [1]. It writes:

$$\frac{\partial u}{\partial t} = \text{div}\,(D\nabla u) + f(u) - v,$$
$$\frac{\partial v}{\partial t} = \epsilon\,(ku - v). \tag{1}$$

where u represents the transmembrane potential and v is an auxiliary variable, and $f(u) = f_0\,u(1-u)(u-a)$. The system is subject to the boundary condition:

$$u(x,t) = e(x,t) \quad x \in \partial\Omega^{\text{Purkinje}},$$

where e is the pulse-shaped input signal.

Anisotropic behaviour is accounted for by making the diffusion matrix D depend on the fibre orientation: $\forall x,\ D(x)\ =\ diag(d, \varepsilon, \varepsilon)$ in the orthonormal basis $(\underline{n}, \underline{k}, \underline{l})$ local to x ; where $\underline{n}$ is a unit vector tangent to the fibre.

The theoretical aspects of (1) have been widely studied [16]: a travelling wave of fixed shape and speed either appears or not, depending on the initial excitation being above or below a threshold. The important parameters are

- a which controls the value of the threshold for excitation;
- D and f_0 which adjust the wave speed and time scale.

A simple output, the electrocardiogram along the axis d, can be calculated as follows:

$$\mathrm{ecg}(d,\ t)\ =\ L(\nabla u(t),\ d).$$

L is a weighted integral over the volume of the heart.

Although more accurate models exist [1], we retained this one, as it correctly captures in a simple formulation, the qualitative behaviour of the wave and leads to fast three dimensional computations [14,10,7,13]. This model would likely be improved by introducing an additional variable [8].

Solutions to (1) have been approximated by using a standard $P1$ Lagrange finite element procedure (with mass lumping and first order numerical integration at vertices), on the given tetrahedral anatomical mesh. Since the time-dependent phenomenon is of interest, small time-steps are used in an explicit procedure (Euler method).

The parameters a, ϵ, k, f_0 are estimated according to the results in [8].

Potential maps such as those illustrated on Figure 1 are derived at different time steps, starting after a wave has been initiated at the apex and propagated. Better initiation points will be chosen according to data from [5].

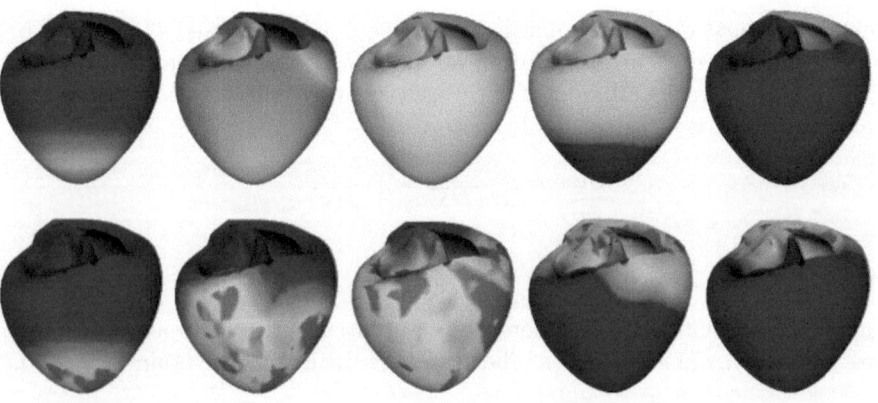

Fig. 1. (Top) Isotropic propagation ($d = 1,\ \varepsilon = 1$), (Bottom) Anisotropic propagation ($d = 1,\ \varepsilon = 0.7$)

This time-dependent computed potential can then be used as an excitation entry to the system describing the mechanical behaviour of the myocardium. No particular feedback is currently used, as proposed in [8] to strengthen the coupling between the electrical and mechanical models.

4   Mechanical Model

The constitutive law that we consider for the cardiac muscle (composed of a distribution of stacked myocardial fibres) is based on the classical Hill-Maxwell rheological model [6], schematically represented in Figure 2 where E_c, E_s and E_p symbolically denote the contractile, series and parallel element, respectively.

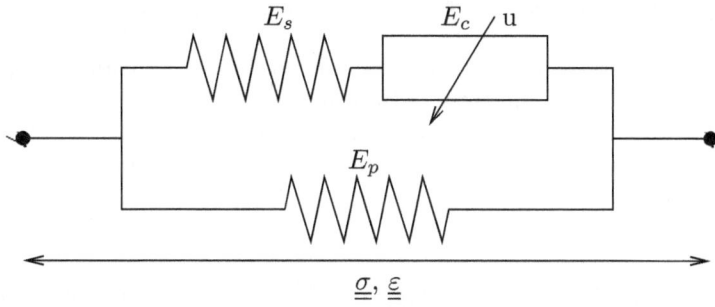

Fig. 2. Hill-Maxwell rheological model

The series and parallel elements are elastic, but non-necessarily linear. The contractile element develops an action oriented in the direction of the fibre at the point in consideration, hence the corresponding stress tensor is everywhere one-dimensional (1D) and in the form $\underline{\underline{\sigma}}_c = \sigma_c\,\underline{n} \otimes \underline{n}$, where $\underline{n}$ denotes the unit vector tangent to the fibre. This implies that the stress tensor corresponding to the series element is also 1D, since $\underline{\underline{\sigma}}_s = \underline{\underline{\sigma}}_c$. In the parallel element, the stress tensor is fully 3D (even though the corresponding constitutive law is strongly anisotropic due to the fibre architecture), so is the global stress tensor given by $\underline{\underline{\sigma}} = \underline{\underline{\sigma}}_c + \underline{\underline{\sigma}}_p$.

For the (scalar) stress quantity σ_c we use a (time-dependent) constitutive relation recently proposed and justified in [3] (see also [4]), viz:

$$\dot{\tilde{\sigma}}_c = -\left(|\dot{\varepsilon}_c| + d|u|\right)\tilde{\sigma}_c + k_c\dot{\varepsilon}_c + \sigma_0|u|_+,$$
$$\dot{k}_c = -\left(|\dot{\varepsilon}_c| + d|u|\right)k_c + k_0|u|_+,$$
$$\sigma_c = k_c\varepsilon_0 + \tilde{\sigma}_c + \nu\dot{\varepsilon}_c.$$

Here, ε_c denotes the (1D) strain corresponding to the contractile element, k_c and $\tilde{\sigma}_c$ represent additional internal variables, u is the input (also represented in

Fig. 2), and all other quantities are constants. The input u is a chemical quantity that depends mainly on the calcium concentration [4], and which is modelled in section 3. Hence, the resulting constitutive law for the global rheological model is of the form $\underline{\underline{\sigma}} = \Sigma\,(\underline{\underline{\varepsilon}}, u)$, where Σ denotes a functional. This constitutive law is then used in combination with the equations of solid dynamics to obtain the mechanical model.

5   Interaction with Ultrasound Images

In our current implementation, we simplify the mechanical model into anisotropic linear elasticity and the fibres activation is modelled as a stress tensor $\sigma_a = \alpha\, f \otimes f$, where α is the activation rate which is directly related to the potential u of Section 3, and f the fibre direction. It gives a force $\mathbf{F}_a$:

$$\mathbf{F}_a = \int_V \mathrm{div}(\sigma_a)\, dv = \int_V \mathrm{div}(\alpha f \otimes f)\, dv = \int_S (\alpha f \otimes f)\,\overline{\otimes}\, n\, ds.$$

Therefore, when a fibre is activated, its contraction is equivalent to a pressure applied to the surface of the tetrahedron in the fibre direction.

Figure 3 presents the results of a contraction proportional to the potential (which should be replaced by a differential equation controlling the activation from the potential).

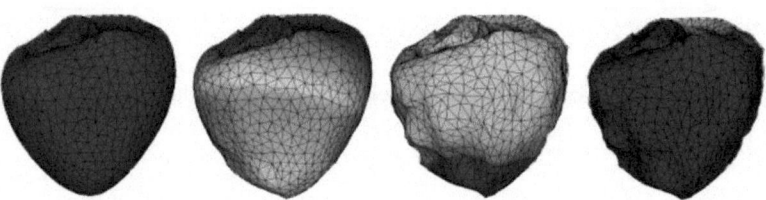

Fig. 3. Effect of the fibres contraction on the 3D model.

The model is also constrained by the ultrasound images (see Fig. 4) through the external forces $\mathbf{F}_i$ which are proportional to the distance to the closest boundary point of the image from the considered point of the mesh.

We use mass-lumping in a Newtonian differential equation with an explicit integration scheme to compute the position $\mathbf{P}$ of each vertex:

$$\left(\frac{1}{\Delta t^2} - \frac{\gamma}{2\Delta t}\right)\mathbf{P}^{t+1} = \mathbf{F}_i + \mathbf{F}_a + \mathbf{F} + \frac{2}{\Delta t^2}\mathbf{P}^t - \left(\frac{1}{\Delta t^2} + \frac{\gamma}{2\Delta t}\right)\mathbf{P}^{t-1},$$

with γ the damping factor. $\mathbf{F}$ represents the forces computed from linear elasticity plus the boundary conditions (in particular the ventricular pressures). As ultrasound data is sparse and noisy, it is efficient to use a volumetric model [11, 12] together with electro-mechanical knowledge to extract information (see [15] for preliminary results).

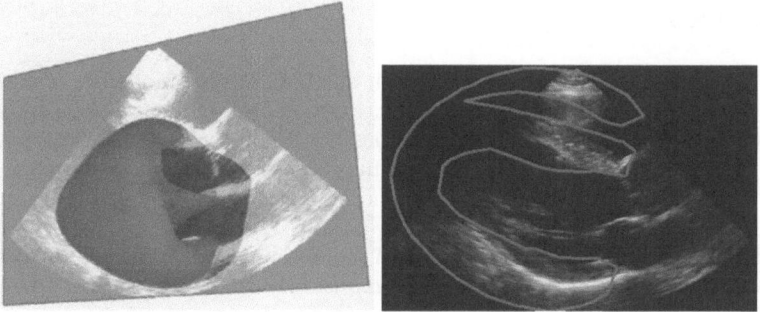

Fig. 4. Left: the 3D model in a slice of the 3D ultrasound image. Right: intersection of the model and the image.

6   Perspectives

Each part of our model is planned to be improved:

- the anatomical model (Section 2) should be based on a human heart. Diffusion MRI is probably one possible way to obtain fibre directions and maybe Purkinje network;
- the electrical model (Section 3) could include a third variable to better control the shape of the wave and a mechano-electrical feedback;
- the mechanical model (Section 4) has to be solved on a 3D mesh;
- the simplified model for ultrasound segmentation (Section 5) will become non-linear.

For each of these models we intend to identify parameters:

- for the electrical parameters, D, f_0, and the electrical entries, Purkinje fibres, ectopic foci, should be estimated by comparing computed ECGs with measured ones. To achieve this, an inverse problem has to be considered;
- for the mechanical parameters, identification techniques still have to be developed, as in vivo rheological studies for human tissues are hard to set up. Here, a criterion will be the difference between the computed motion and the one extracted from the ultrasound images.

All these points will be the topics of our future work.

Acknowledgements. This work was partially funded by the scientific direction of INRIA through a Collaborative Research Action called ICEMA[1] involving the INRIA research groups Epidaure, Macs, Sinus, Sosso and PRF (Philips Research France).

The cardiac mesh data and fibre direction were provided by the University of Auckland, New Zealand[2].

---

[1] http://www-rocq.inria.fr/ frclemen/icema.html
[2] http://www.esc.auckland.ac.nz/Groups/Bioengineering/

References

1. A.L. Bardou, P.M. Auger, P.J. Birkui, and J.L. Chass. Modeling of cardiac electrophysiological mechanisms: From action potential genesis to its propagation in myocardium. *Critical Reviews in Biomedical Engineering*, 24:141–221, 1996.
2. O. Berenfeld and J. Jalife. Purkinje-muscle rentry as a mechanism of polymorphic ventricular arrhytmias in a 3-dimensional model of the ventricles. *Circ. Res.*, 82:1063–1077, 1998.
3. J. Bestel, F. Clément, and M. Sorine. A biomechanical model of muscle contraction. In *Medical Image Computing and Computer-Assisted intervention (MICCAI'01)*, 2001.
4. J. Bestel and M. Sorine. A differential model of muscle contraction and applications. In *Schlœssman Seminar on Mathematical Models in Biology, Chenistry and Physics*, 2000.
5. D. Durrer, R.T. van Dam, G.E Freud, M.J. Janse, F.L. Miejler, and R.C. Arzbaecher. Total excitation of the isolated human heart. *Circulation*, 41:899–912, 1970.
6. A.V. Hill. The heat of shortening and the dynamic constants in muscle. *Proc. Roy. Soc. London*, 126:136–165, 1938.
7. A.V. Holden and A.V. Panfilov. *Computational biology of the heart*, chapter Modelling propagation in excitable media, pages 65–99. John Wiley & Sons, 1996.
8. Z. Knudsen, A.V. Holden, and J. Brindley. Qualitative modelling of mechano electrical feedback in a ventricular cell. *Bulletin of mathematical biology*, 6(59):115–181, 1997.
9. M. Nash. *Mechanics and Material Properties of the Heart using an Anatomically Accurate Mathematical Model*. PhD thesis, University ofAuckland, 1998.
10. A.V. Panfilov and A.V. Holden. Computer-simulation of reentry sources in myocardium in 2 and 3 dimensions. *Journal of Theoretical Biology*, 3(161):271–285, 1993.
11. X. Papademetris, A.J. Sinusas, D.P. Dione, and J.S. Duncan. Estimation of 3D left ventricle deformation from echocardiography. *Medical Image Analysis*, 5(1):17–28, 2001.
12. Q.C. Pham, F. Vincent, P. Clarysse, P. Croisille, and I. Magnin. A FEM-based deformable model for the 3D segmentation and tracking of the heart in cardiac mri. In *Image and Signal Processing and Analysis (ISPA'01)*, 2001.
13. A.E. Pollard, N. Hooke, and C.S. Henriquez. Cardiac propagation simulation. *Critical Reviews in biomedical Engineering*, 20(3,4):171–210, 1992.
14. J. Rogers, M. Courtemanche, and A. McCulloch. *Computational biology of the heart*, chapter Finite element methods for modelling impulse propagation in the heart, pages 217–233. John Wiley & Sons, 1996.
15. M. Sermesant, Y. Coudière, H. Delingette, N. Ayache, and J.A. Désidéri. An electro-mechanical model of the heart for cardiac image segmentation. In *Medical Image Computing and Computer-Assisted intervention (MICCAI'01)*, 2001.
16. J. Smoller. *Shock Waves and Reaction-Diffusion Equations*. Springer-Verlag (Grundlehren der mathematischen Wissenschaften 258), 1983.

A Physiologically-Based Model for the Active Cardiac Muscle Contraction

Dominique Chapelle, Frédérique Clément, Frank Génot,
Patrick Le Tallec, Michel Sorine, and José M. Urquiza

INRIA-Rocquencourt, BP 105, 78153 Le Chesnay, France,
Dominique.Chapelle@inria.fr

Abstract. We present a 3D mechanical model for the behaviour of the cardiac muscle, based on a recently proposed model of myofibre contraction. The construction of the 3D model involves a rheological model similar to that of Hill-Maxwell. We then introduce some discretisation techniques adapted to our mechanical model, and we report on some preliminary numerical results.

1 Introduction

Like most biological materials, the cardiac muscle displays strongly nonlinear and anisotropic mechanical behaviour, see, e.g., [5]. Anisotropy is governed—in particular—by the architecture of muscle fibres and of the fibre sheets. Moreover, muscle fibres are responsible for the active stress generated by the electrical stimulations. This active stress mainly concerns the stress component along the fibre direction, which is also the primary direction of electrical propagation.

In this work we present a complete mechanical model that aims at correctly representing the cardiac muscle behaviour in the presence of the chemical/electrical stimulation. This model is based on a recently proposed myofibre model [2], which we recall before presenting the methodology allowing its incorporation into a global three-dimensional (3D) mechanical model. The last section is devoted to numerical discretisation strategies adapted to the model, and we present some preliminary numerical results obtained for a 1D simplified problem.

2 The Excitation-Contraction Myofibre Model

The myofibre model introduced and justified in [2] (see also [3]), is based on the classical Hill-Maxwell rheological model [6], depicted in Figure 1. Elastic material laws are used for the series element E_s and for the parallel element E_p. Based on empirical results, the corresponding stress-strain laws are generally assumed to be of exponential type [9,12].

The element E_c accounts for the contractile electrically-activated part of the behaviour. In order to represent this behaviour, we use the constitutive law

T. Katila et al. (Eds.): FIMH 2001, LNCS 2230, pp. 128–133, 2001.

recently proposed in [2] (a refinement of the model presented in [3]), based on the microstructural *sliding filament* model of Huxley [8] and the *distribution-moment* approach of Zahalak [13]. This (time-dependent) constitutive law reads

$$\begin{cases} \dot{\tilde{\sigma}}_c = -(|\dot{\varepsilon}_c| + |u|), \tilde{\sigma}_c + k_c \dot{\varepsilon}_c + \sigma_0 |u|_+, \\ \dot{k}_c = -(|\dot{\varepsilon}_c| + |u|)k_c + k_0 |u|_+ \\ \sigma_c = k_c \varepsilon_0 + \tilde{\sigma}_c + \nu \dot{\varepsilon}_c, \end{cases} \tag{1}$$

where u is the excitation, a chemical quantity that mainly depends on the calcium concentration, $\dot{\varepsilon}_c$ stands for the time derivative of ε_c, and σ_0, k_0, ε_0, ν are local parameters such that σ_0, k_0, $\nu > 0$. This model is also in accordance with observations made on the passive behaviour of the muscle [10].

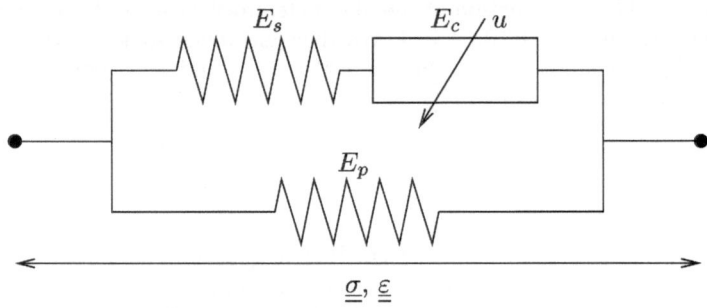

Fig. 1. Hill-Maxwell rheological model

3   Geometry, Fibre Orientations, and Governing Equations of Activated Heart Contractions

In order to construct our global 3D mechanical model we need:

- Anatomical data allowing for a definition of the heart geometry, with an accurate description of the microstructural anatomy, i.e. of the orientations of muscle fibres and fibre sheets.
- The governing equations of the 3D mechanical behaviour.

We used the anatomical data provided by the Auckland biomedical engineering research group [7]. We refined the original mesh composed of hexahedral elements by using the softwares YAMS and GHS3D developped at INRIA in the Gamma team [4,11]. The refined mesh, composed of tetrahedral elements, is shown in Figure 2.

The orientation of the fibres is available at each integration point in the mesh. The corresponding streamline representation is shown in Figure 3.

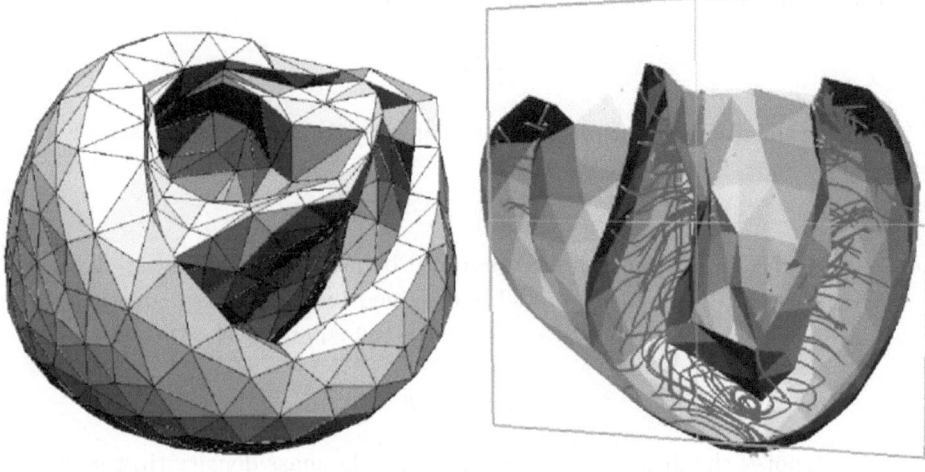

Fig. 2. Refined tetrahedral mesh   **Fig. 3.** Heart fibre directions

We now introduce the governing 3D mechanical equations. We denote by $\underline{F}$ and $\underline{\underline{\varepsilon}}$ the deformation gradient and the Green-Lagrange strain tensor, respectively. We then use the second Piola-Kirchhoff stress tensor, denoted by $\underline{\underline{\sigma}}$. Recalling the rheological model of Figure 1, the total stress is the sum of the stresses in the two branches. The branch containing the contractile element, however, only contributes to the stress tensor in the direction of the fibre, given by the unit tangent vector $\underline{n}$. Namely, we have

$$\underline{\underline{\sigma}} = \underline{\underline{\sigma}}_p + \sigma_{1D}\,\underline{n} \otimes \underline{n}, \tag{2}$$

where σ_{1D} is a scalar quantity that represents the (second Piola-Kirchhoff) stress in the series branch. The series kinematics and the one-dimensional character of the deformation in this branch imply that the corresponding (scalar) Green-Lagrange strain

$$\varepsilon_{1D} = \sum_{i,j} \varepsilon_{ij} n_i n_j \tag{3}$$

satisfies the multiplicative law

$$1 + \varepsilon_{1D} = (1 + \varepsilon_c)(1 + \varepsilon_s), \tag{4}$$

where ε_c and ε_s denote the strains in the contractile and series element, respectively (note that this relation reduces to the usual additive law in the case of small strains). Furthermore, the associated second Piola-Kirchhoff stresses satisfy, by formal thermodynamical considerations,

$$\sigma_{1D} = \frac{\sigma_c}{1 + \varepsilon_s} = \frac{\sigma_s}{1 + \varepsilon_c}. \tag{5}$$

On the other hand, the parallel kinematics directly implies

$$\underline{\underline{\varepsilon}} = \underline{\underline{\varepsilon}}_p. \tag{6}$$

Combining the above equations with the constitutive laws of the elastic elements

$$\sigma_s = \sigma_s(\varepsilon_s), \qquad \underline{\underline{\sigma}}_p = \underline{\underline{\sigma}}_p(\underline{\underline{\varepsilon}}_p), \tag{7}$$

and with the equations (1), the 3D material behaviour is completely defined.

The global 3D mechanical model is obtained by using these constitutive relations (involving the input u) together with the equation of dynamics

$$\mathrm{div}(\underline{\underline{F}} \cdot \underline{\underline{\sigma}}) - \rho \underline{\ddot{y}} = \underline{0}, \tag{8}$$

where $\underline{y}$ denotes the displacement vector and ρ the mass density (in the original configuration).

4   A One-Dimensional Activated Fibre Contraction

As a model problem we consider a one-dimensional homogeneous medium governed by a 1D reduction of equations (1)-(8).

In this first step to the numerical exploration of the excitation-contraction model we use the infinitesimal displacement assumption: with $y(x,t)$ denoting the longitudinal displacement of a material point located at position x, $0 < x < 1$, in a reference stress-free state, the deformation is given by $\varepsilon(x,t) = \frac{\partial y(x,t)}{\partial x}$. Moreover, we assume that series and parallel elements are linear and that $\nu = 0$, $\varepsilon_0 = 0$. The considered equations read

$$\begin{cases} \rho \ddot{y} - \frac{\partial}{\partial x}(k_p \varepsilon + \sigma_c) = 0, \\ \dot{\sigma}_c = -(|\dot{\varepsilon}_c| + |u|)\sigma_c + k_c \dot{\varepsilon}_c + \sigma_0 |u|_+, \\ \dot{k}_c = -(|\dot{\varepsilon}_c| + |u|)k_c + k_0 |u|_+, \\ \sigma_c = k_s(\varepsilon - \varepsilon_c), \end{cases} \tag{9}$$

with positive constants k_p and k_s. We also consider that the body is fixed at both ends, that is $y(0,t) = y(1,t) = 0$, corresponding to an isometric contraction or relaxation.

Performing a variational finite element space discretization with piecewise-linear continuous functions for the displacement and piecewise-constant functions for stress and deformation variables, we use a midpoint scheme for solving the resulting system of differential-algebraic equations (see [1]).

In the numerical tests presented in Figures 4 to 7 we chose all initial unknowns to be zero. These numerical experiments illustrate the active contraction (positive u) and active relaxation (negative u) abilities of the model.

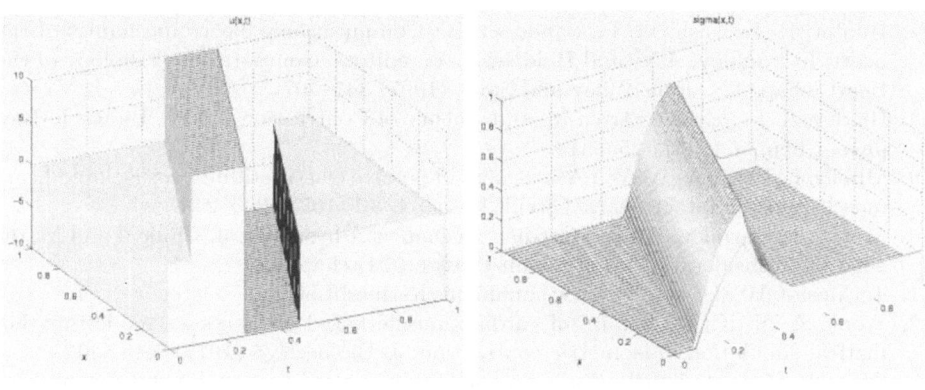

Fig. 4. Electric excitation   **Fig. 5.** Resulting stress

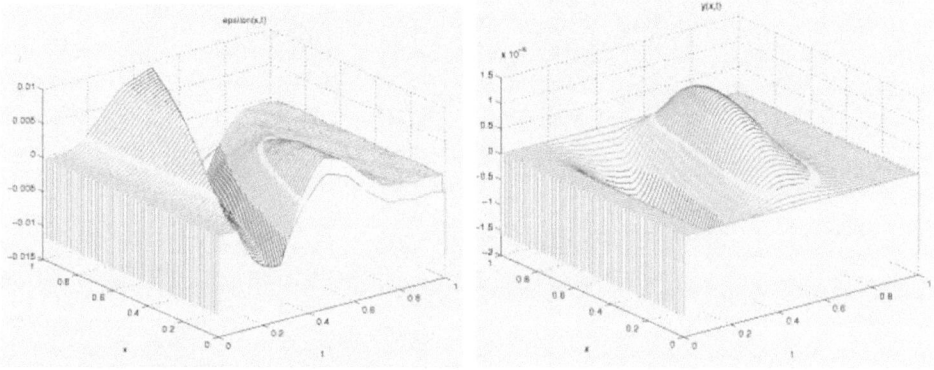

Fig. 6. Deformation   **Fig. 7.** Displacement

References

1. Ascher, U. M., Petzold, L. M.: Computer Methods for Ordinary Differential Equations and Differential-Algebraic Equations. SIAM Publ., Philadelphia (1998)
2. Bestel, J., Clément F., Sorine, M.: A biomechanical model of muscle contraction. Fourth Int. Conf. on Medical Image Computing and Computer-Assisted Intervention, Utrecht, The Netherlands (2001)
3. Bestel, J., Sorine, M.: A differential model of muscle contraction and applications. Schlœssman Seminar on Mathematical Models in Biology, Chemistry and Physics Max Planck Society, Bad Lausick, Germany (2000)
4. Frey, P. J., Borouchaki, H.: Geometric surface mesh optimization. Comput. Visual. in Science **1** (1998) 113–121
5. Fung, Y. C.: Biomechanics: Mechanical Properties of Living Tissues. Springer-Verlag, 2nd Ed. (1993)
6. Hill, A. V.: The heat of shortening and the dynamic constants in muscle. Proc. Roy. Soc. London (B) **126** (1938) 136–195

7. Hunter, P. J., Nash, M. P., Sands, G. B.: Computational electromechanics of the heart. In Panfilov, A.V. and Holden, A. V., editors, Computational Biology of the Heart, chap. 12 , John Wiley and Sons, (1997) 345–407
8. Huxley, A. F.: Muscle Structure and Theory of Contraction. Progr. Biomech. Biophys. Chem. **7** (1957) 255–318
9. Mirsky, I., Parmley, W. W.: Assessment of passive elastic stiffness for isolated heart muscle and the intact heart. Circul. Research **33** (1973) 233–243
10. Mirsky, I., Parmley, W. W.: Cardiac Mechanics: Physiological, Clinical and Mathematical Considerations. Pergamon Press (1974) chap. 4
11. TetMesh-GHS3D: http://www.simulog.fr/itetmeshf.htm
12. Wong, A. Y. K.: Mechanics of cardiac muscle based on Huxley's model: mathematical simulation of isometric contraction. J. Biomech. **4** (1971) 529–540
13. Zahalak, G. I.: A distribution-moment approximation for kinetic theories of muscular contraction. Math. Biosci. **55** (1981) 89–114

Post-Systolic Thickening in Ischaemic Myocardium: A Simple Mathematical Model for Simulating Regional Deformation

Piet Claus, Bart Bijnens, Frank Weidemann, Christoph Dommke,
Virginie Bito, Frank Heinzel, Karin Sipido, Ivan De Scheerder,
Frank E. Rademakers, and George R. Sutherland

Department of Cardiology, K.U. Leuven, University Hospitals Gasthuisberg,
Herestraat 49, B–3000 Leuven, Belgium
Piet.Claus@uz.kuleuven.ac.be

Abstract. We present a one-dimensional mathematical model to explain changes in regional radial myocardial deformation during ischaemia. The model makes use of cellular contraction properties of normal and ischaemic myocytes extracted from an animal model of induced chronic, regional ischaemia of the posterior wall. Simulations of the model are compared to the deformation patterns observed in the experimental animal models of regional ischaemia.

1 Introduction

Localized, regional ischaemia induces reduced systolic thickening with a concomitant increase in post-systolic thickening (PST). Prior experimental and clinical observations proposed acute development and presence of PST in an ischaemic myocardial segment as a potential marker of myocardial viability. With the introduction of (echocardiographic) strain and strain rate imaging as a new clinical tool to non-invasively quantify regional myocardial deformation [1], evaluating explicit markers such as PST can increase the clinical potential of the method. Controlled experimental work, e.g. [2,3,4,5], has shown a complex mechanical behaviour of the ischaemic myocardium. In summary in ischaemic myocardium the following observations can be made: (a) during the isovolumetric contraction period and early systole, myocardial thinning occurs, (b) in systole, the magnitude of regional thickening/shortening is decreased, (c) after aortic valve closure, normal relaxation and thinning (lengthening) is interchanged with ongoing post-systolic thickening (shortening). The magnitude of these alterations is proportional to the severity of the ischaemic insult. This phenomenon occurs in acute, prolonged as well as in chronic regional ischaemia. Despite the multitude of experimental work, the mechanisms underlying PST remain unclear. The debate is still going on whether this phenomenon is active, i.e. the thickening in the ischaemic segment is due to late, prolonged contraction in the ischaemic fibres, or passive, thickening due to the elastic force from the interaction between the relaxing normal segments and the ischaemic segment. In this paper,

T. Katila et al. (Eds.): FIMH 2001, LNCS 2230, pp. 134–139, 2001.
© Springer-Verlag Berlin Heidelberg 2001

we try to make a further step in the explanation of this phenomenon. Assuming that PST mostly depends on regional heterogeneity in contractile and/or elastic properties of interacting segments of myocardium, we have developed a simple one-dimensional model reflecting these properties, which explains these phenomena, at least qualitatively.

2 Theoretical Model

In this section we present a simple model of normal and ischaemic myocardium, interacting during a cardiac cycle.

2.1 Description

Though, anatomically accurate models have been constructed for the heart, we will rely on a simplified model, using finite difference techniques to solve the dynamics. Despite the fact that this model has severe limitations, it is able to simulate qualitatively the regional deformation patterns of the myocardium. The choice of the simple model enables us to solve the equations of motion for the nodes in fig. 1 straightforwardly, by simple time step integration techniques, in a limited computation time ($\pm 50s$), using Matlab (The MathWorks, Inc.).
Model geometry. In the model a midwall segment of the left ventricle is effectively described by a discretised, closed chain where the thickness of the wall is defined as a field on this chain. The reduction from the three dimensional structure to the one-dimensional model is depicted in Fig. 1. This effective model takes out the interactions in the longitudinal directions of the left-ventricular wall. The

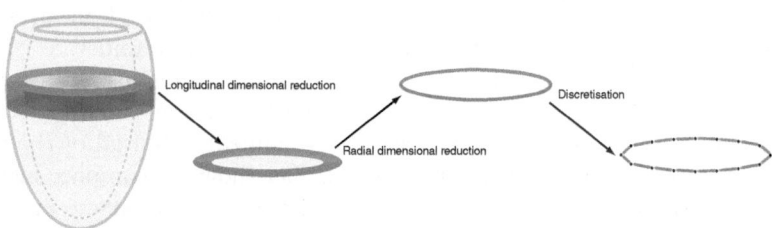

Fig. 1. Representation of the reduction steps from a mid-wall slice of myocardium to the discrete one-dimensional description (red:ischaemic, blue:normal)

model allows for a connected variable sized region of ischeamic segments along the chain. The "thickness"of the elements is defined to be proportional to the reciprocal of the length of the elements (based on local mass conservation). In fig. 1, half of the chain is ischaemic and half is normal. The elements are described as Maxwell elements splitting active and passive properties of the elements. It describes the element as a contractile component (CE) in series with an elastic component (SE), together in parallel with another elastic component (PE).

136   P. Claus et al.

Passive elastic properties. The SE and PE are described as non-linear springs, with a passive length-tension relation, i.e.

$$T = C/K(e^{K\lambda(t)} - 1)\,, \qquad \text{where} \qquad \lambda = \frac{l - l_0}{l_0}\,. \tag{1}$$

$l(t)$ is the instantaneous length and l_0 the end-diastolic length of the segments. The parallel component of the Maxwell elements is assumed to take into account the elasticity of the extracellular collagen matrix.

Active properties. The active developed contraction force of the segments is modeled by a gaussian, with variable amplitude and width, which can be shifted in time, allowing variation of the amplitude, duration and onset of the active contraction. Again, this is an extensive simplification of the active contraction sequence. Complete models includes a large number of parameters and state variables, which leads to a better representation but also decrease the possibility of estimating parameters from them.

Boundary Conditions. As a boundary condition the intercavitary pressure was simulated according to measured pressure curves (fig. 3).

2.2   Simulations

To simulate the radial deformation during a complete cardiac cycle, the cycle was divided into 800 time steps of 1 ms. We divided the cycle into 4 events, isovolumetric contraction period (0–50ms) (end: aortic valve opening), ejection (50–300ms) (end: aortic valve closure), isovolumetric relaxation period (300–350ms) (end: mitral valve closure) and diastole (350–800ms) (end: mitral valve opening). Equations of motion were integrated at each time step. The chain was divided into 50 segments/nodes and had a diastolic radius of 2 cm, corresponding to an average diastolic cavity radius of the pig model of section 3.

During the isovolumetric periods motion of the nodes perpendicular to the instantaneous segment directions was restricted. This perpendicular motion was not restricted to zero because deformation and motion caused by shape changes can occur during the isovolumetric periods.

The final result of the simulations was the natural transmural radial strain, which represents wall-thickening during the heart cycle.

We have performed three groups of simulations to study myocardial ischaemia: reduced perfusion, total occlusion and infarction. For reduced perfusion and total occlusion, the passive properties of the ischemic zone were taken to be normal, but in the case of reduced perfusion, the active contraction force was prolonged and reduced, in accordance with the results of cellular contraction measurements from the experimental pig model, (see section 3). For total occlusion the active force equals zero. Infarction was simulated by zero active force, but with higher stiffness constants in the ischaemic zone. The qualitative simulation results for radial strain are summarized in fig. 2.

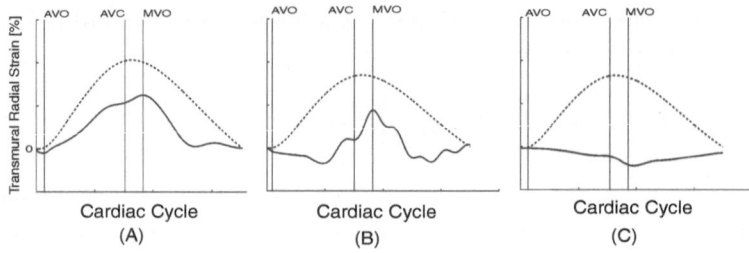

Fig. 2. Simulation results. (A)Reduced perfusion. (B)Total occlusion. (C)Infarction. Dashed line: Radial strain in the middel segment of the normal zone, Solid line: Radial strain in the middle segment of the ischaemic zone. AVC: Aortic valve closure, MVO: Mitral valve opening.

3   Comparison of the Model with Experimental Data

In this section we shortly describe a pig model for induced regional chronic ischaemia and present some data. This closed chest model was developed to get a spectrum of chronic regional ischaemia, reflecting the clinical setting. The

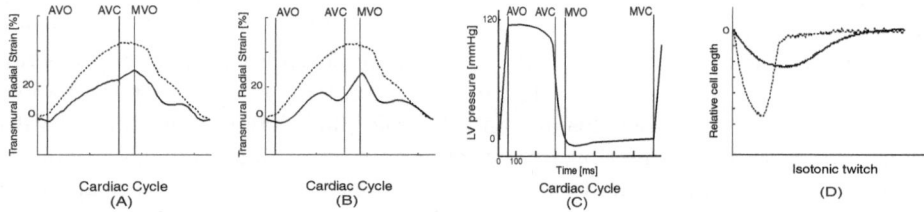

Fig. 3. Experimental data. (A)Transmural radial strain (wall thickening) curves from the chronic ischaemic posterior wall of the pig model, (B) Transmural radial strain curve from a pig experiment of acute total occlusion [5]. (C)Pressure curve measured in experiment and used as boundary condition for simulations. (D)Single twitches from stimulated single cells (dashed: normal myocytes, solid: ischaemic myocytes). AVO/AVC: Aortic valve opening/closure, MVO/MVC: Mitral valve opening/closure.

model has been developed, by implanting a copper coated stent in the proximal segment of the left circumflex coronary artery. Two weeks after implantation the percent diameter of the developed stenosis was estimated by angiography and ultrasound strain rate imaging was performed according to the protocol described in [5]. After sacrifice of the pigs the heart was taken out and prepared for cell extraction. The radial strain curves of the posterior wall are depicted in fig. 3(A). Cells of the ischaemic region of the excised heart were isolated and compared with cells of the same region of normal hearts. Cell contraction in isotonic twitches of single cells have been measured and are depicted in Fig. 3(D).

4   Discussion

The proposed simple one-dimensional model is able to simulate the regional radial deformation curves for a whole spectrum of ischaemic myocardium, as observed in diverse experimental settings [4,5]. The model is based on only a small number of parameters for normal and ischaemic regions, i.e. elasticity constants together with strength, length and onset of actively developed force. From the close resemblance between measured and simulated deformations we can infer that these are the major determinants of the observed phenomena.

One of the major objectives of the simulation study was to get insight into the physiological mechanisms behind PST, an abberant myocardial thickening, occuring in what is traditionally perceived as the relaxation (and thus thining) phase of the cardiac cycle. Two different explanations have been proposed, namely "active" and "passive" thickening. Active thickening after aortic valve closure could occur if there is a delayed and/or prolonged active contraction force developed in the myocytes. On the other hand, passive thickening could be explained by the interaction with neighbouring segments. In this hypothesis, ischaemic tissue would not thicken by itself, but exhibits a pulling force from the neighbouring thickening (normal) myocardium. Since, before aortic closure, pressure is high in the cavity, this pulling force is not sufficient to deform the non-contracting part as much as the normal tissue, resulting in less deformation (explaining the observed decrease in systolic thickening). However, after the sudden drop in pressure associated with aortic valve closure, the pulling force from the normal (and at that moment thicker) tissue can further deform the ischaemic region, until the dimensions are similar to the (at that moment thining) normal neighbouring part. This would explain the observed PST.

The implemented model was developed in such a way that both hypotheses could be investigated. Therefore, elastic properties and myocyte contraction parameters (for the actively developed forces) were combined.

To investigate whether the *passive theory* could completely explain PST in all cases, a total occlusion simulation, i.e. no active force is present, was performed (Fig. 2(B)). When comparing findings with experimental total occlusion (Fig. 3(B)), the observed deformation patterns are very similar, confirming the *passive* explanation. Also, when tissue elasticity is decreased in the model , mimicking the development of fibrosis after infarction, myocardial strain could be predicted by the simulation (Fig. 2(C)), solely based on *passive* phenomena.

However, strain curves, measured during experimental reduced perfusion, cannot be explained by the model when only incorporating passive deformation. From the experiments in isolated myocytes, we could observe that in chronic ischaemia there is a prolonged, but reduced contraction of the cells, with no delay in onset. Consequently, this observation was used as input for further simulations. Fig. 2(A) shows the result of the simulation where, additionally to the *passive* interaction of segments, a reduced and prolonged contraction force was imposed on the ischaemic region. Under these conditions, it can be clearly observed when comparing to the measured strain curves in case of experimentally reduced perfusion (Fig. 3(A)), that this combination of the *passive* and *active* hypotheses explains both the systolic and the post-systolic deformation of ischaemic myocardium.

Additionally, in all cases, the simulations exhibited early thinning of the ischaemic segments. During the isovolumetric contraction period the segments can rearrange in the circumferential directions. During this early period in the cardiac cycle, the normal segments develop a higher contraction force and stretch the ischaemic segments, which results in a temporary thinning.

As a conclusion, we can state that our model would support the following hypothesis regarding myocardial deformation during ischaemia: With decreasing coronary flow, there is a decrease in systolic thickening caused by a reduction of the *active* contraction force developed in the myocytes. After aortic valve closure, there is a further thickening (PST) where a contineous thickening is caused by a delayed *active* contraction and sudden changes in thickness can be explained by *passive* interaction with surrounding tissue, after all active force development ceased. The more the perfusion is diminished, the more the deformation will be governed by *passive* mechanisms.

Finally, we remark that although the model explains qualitatively the mechanisms of PST, it has its limitations. It does not take into account longitudinal deformation. Additionally, in the diastolic phase the model can not explain the biphasic responses of the radial strain. In part this is due to the fact that we take the overall pressure as the external force that act on the myocardium, while in reality this strain is influenced by the propagation of the pressure wave and its associated vortices. Therefore, quantitative results from the model cannot be trusted.

References

1. J. D'hooge, A. Heimdal, F. Jamal, T. Kukulski, B. Bijnens, F. Rademakers, L. Hatle, P. Suetens and G.R. Sutherland: Regional Strain and Strain rate Measurements by Cardiac Ultrasound: Principles, Implementation and Limitations. Eur. J. Echocardiography **1** (2000) 154–170.
2. P. Theroux, D. Franklin, J. Ross, and W.S. Qemper: Regional myocardial function during acute coronary artery occlusion and its modification by pharmacologic agent in the dog. Circ. Res. **35** (1974) 896–908.
3. B.J. Leone, R.M. Norris, A. Safwat, P Foqx and W.A. Ryder: Effects of progressive myocardial ischaemia on systolic function, diastolic function, and load dependent relaxation. Circ. Res. **26** (1992) 422-429.
4. T. Ihara, K. Komamura,Y.T. Shen, T.A. Patrick, I. Mirsky, R.P. Shannon and S.F. Vatner, Left ventricular systolic dysfunction and precedes diastolic dysfunction during myocardial ischemia in concious dogs. Am. J. Physiol. **267** (1994) H333–H343.
5. F. Jamal, T. Kukulski, J. Strotmann, M. Szilard, J. D'hooge, B. Bijnens,F. Rademakers, L. Hatle, I. De Scheerder and G.R. Sutherland Quantitation of the Spectrum of Changes in Regional Myocardial Function During Acute Ischaemia in Closed-Chest Pigs. An Ultrasonic Strain Rate and Strain Study, J Am. Soc. Echocardiography, in press 2001.

Simulation of Anisotropic Propagation in the Myocardium with a Hybrid Bidomain Model

Kim Simelius[1], Jukka Nenonen[1], and B. Milan Horáček[2]

[1] Helsinki University of Technology, Laboratory of Biomedical Engineering,
P.O. Box 2200, 02015 HUT, Finland
(Kim.Simelius, Jukka.Nenonen)@hut.fi
http://www.hut.fi/Units/Biomedical
[2] Dalhousie University, Department of Physiology and Biophysics,
Halifax, N.S., Canada
mhoracek@biophy.bp.dal.ca
http://www.physiology.dal.ca

Abstract. We describe simulations of propagated electrical excitation in three-dimensional anisotropic myocardial muscle. According to the bidomain theory, anisotropic electrical conductivities are presented as tensors in the intracellular and interstitial domains (D_i and D_e, respectively). Under the assumption of equal anisotropy ratio ($D_i = kD_e$), subthreshold behaviour of the excitable elements is governed by a parabolic reaction-diffusion equation for the membrane potential, solvable even on a desktop computer. In the case of more general anisotropies ($D_i \neq kD_e$), also the interstitial potential needs to be solved simultaneously from an elliptic partial differential equation, requiring a supercomputer for large arrays of excitable elements. In both cases, the elements obey cellular automata rules in the suprathreshold state. We present preliminary results of the propagated excitation for different anisotropy ratios in a three-dimensional slab geometry.

1   Introduction

First idealized models describing the normal activation sequence in the human heart were reported over two decades ago [1,2,3]. Mainly due to computational limitations, the models did not include myocardial anisotropy nor physiological propagation. On the basis of anisotropic bidomain theory and cellular automata theory, development of more realistic whole-heart models have become feasible. A ventricular model that produces a correct normal activation sequence is a prerequisite for simulating pathological conditions, such as ischemia, infarction or ventricular arrhythmias.

We describe here the theoretical basis of the Dalhousie hybrid propagation model [4,5,6], based on equal anisotropy ratio and cellular automata. We present how the model can be extended to more general anisotropies and show our first simulations in a three-dimensional slab geometry. Due to extensive computational requirements, such simulations may be too demanding to cover the whole ventricles ($\sim 2 \times 10^6$ elements), but they are still useful to explore the validity of the simpler equal anisotropy approach. Furthermore, unequal anisotropy may be necessary to simulate detailed characteristics of the epi- and endocardial potential distributions.

T. Katila et al. (Eds.): FIMH 2001, LNCS 2230, pp. 140–147, 2001.
© Springer-Verlag Berlin Heidelberg 2001

2   Bidomain Theory

The basis of our model is the bidomain theory for anisotropic myocardium, which rests on the assumption that the cardiac tissue functions as an electrically conductive syncytium consisting of two interpenetrating domains—intracellular (i) and interstitial (e)—connected everywhere via the cell membrane [2,3]. Consider the anisotropic bidomain region H, which represents a system of cylindrical myocardial fibers with anisotropic electrical conductivity [7,8]; H is embedded in a bounded, insulated and isotropic conducting medium B. A tissue structure in H is assumed to have *longitudinal* fiber direction defined by a unit vector $\mathbf{a}_\ell(\mathbf{x})$ that is allowed to vary with position $\mathbf{x}$, while intracellular and interstitial domains share the same $\mathbf{a}_\ell(\mathbf{x})$. The local basis consisting of an orthogonal set $\{\mathbf{a}_1(\mathbf{x}), \mathbf{a}_2(\mathbf{x}), \mathbf{a}_3(\mathbf{x})\}$ is chosen at $\mathbf{x}$ so that a unit vector $\mathbf{a}_3(\mathbf{x})$ is parallel with $\mathbf{a}_\ell(\mathbf{x})$; unit vectors $\mathbf{a}_1(\mathbf{x})$ and $\mathbf{a}_2(\mathbf{x})$, and all vectors coplanar with them, are said to be in the *transverse* direction at $\mathbf{x}$. In the local basis, the intracellular conductivities along the axes are $\sigma_1^i, \sigma_2^i, \sigma_3^i$, and the corresponding interstitial conductivities are $\sigma_1^e, \sigma_2^e, \sigma_3^e$; due to axial symmetry of each fiber, $\sigma_1^{i,e} = \sigma_2^{i,e} = \sigma_t^{i,e}$ are conductivities in the transverse direction, and $\sigma_3^{i,e} = \sigma_\ell^{i,e}$ are conductivities in the longitudinal direction. Moreover, uniform anisotropy assumption requires that scalar constants $\sigma_t^{i,e}, \sigma_\ell^{i,e}$ are independent of $\mathbf{x}$.

2.1   Conductivity Tensors

Let us introduce second-rank tensors D_i^* and D_e^* to describe comprehensively the intracellular and interstitial anisotropic conductivities [8]. In the local basis the conductivity tensors are diagonal: $D_{i,e}^* = \mathrm{diag}(\sigma_t^{i,e}, \sigma_t^{i,e}, \sigma_\ell^{i,e})$. To allow variable fiber direction, set the global (cartesian) coordinate system in which local basis is defined at any $\mathbf{x}$ as $A = (\mathbf{a}_1(\mathbf{x}), \mathbf{a}_2(\mathbf{x}), \mathbf{a}_3(\mathbf{x}))$, where $\mathbf{a}_1(\mathbf{x})$, $\mathbf{a}_2(\mathbf{x})$, and $\mathbf{a}_3(\mathbf{x})$ are the column vectors. To represent tensors D_i^* and D_e^* in the global coordinate system, the local basis has to be rotated by multiplying it on each side by a rotation matrix. In the global coordinate system the conductivity tensors are then $D_{i,e} = A D_{i,e}^* A^T$, where the superscript T denotes matrix transpose. Therefore, we can write the conductivity tensors $D_{i,e}$ as [6]

$$D_{i,e} = (\sigma_\ell^{i,e} - \sigma_t^{i,e})\mathbf{a}_\ell \mathbf{a}_\ell^T + \sigma_t^{i,e} I, \qquad (1)$$

where I is the identity matrix. Thus, according to Eq. 1, an anisotropic medium can be thought of as having isotropic conductivities $\sigma_t^{i,e}$ throughout, plus the "boost" in conductivities, $(\sigma_\ell^{i,e} - \sigma_t^{i,e})$, along the fiber direction. In addition to conductivity tensors D_i and D_e, we will introduce a conductivity tensor $D = D_i + D_e$, which will characterize the composite medium of the *bulk* cardiac tissue.

2.2   Electrical Potential Distribution and Current Flow

Electrical potential and current density are defined in H as macroscopic quantities, which may be considered to be averages over small volumes of cardiac tissue encompassing several cells. The current densities are given by the Ohm's law:

$$\mathbf{J}_i = -D_i \nabla \phi_i, \quad \mathbf{J}_e = -D_e \nabla \phi_e \quad \text{in } H,$$

$$\mathbf{J}_o = -\sigma_o \nabla \phi_o \quad \text{in } B, \qquad (2)$$

where ϕ_i and ϕ_e are, respectively, electrical potentials in intracellular and interstitial domains; ϕ_o is the extracardiac potential and σ_o is the isotropic scalar conductivity outside of H. In the bidomain region, the total macroscopic current density, $\mathbf{J}$, is then

$$\mathbf{J} = \mathbf{J}_i + \mathbf{J}_e = -D_i\nabla\phi_i - D_e\nabla\phi_e \quad \text{in } H. \tag{3}$$

It is well established that the electrocardiographic volume-conductor problem can be treated as a quasi-static one [9]. Under the quasi-static assumption, the conservation law requires that the divergence of total current density vanishes ($\nabla \cdot \mathbf{J} = 0$), which leads to

$$\nabla \cdot (D_i\nabla\phi_i + D_e\nabla\phi_e) = 0 \quad \text{in } H, \tag{4}$$

i.e., current can flow from one domain to the other, but there are no net sources or sinks of current in H. Moreover, since thereare no sources in B,

$$\nabla \cdot \mathbf{J}_o = \nabla \cdot \sigma_o\nabla\phi_o = 0 \quad \text{in } B. \tag{5}$$

The intracellular and interstitial domains are coupled through a distributed cellular membrane; the outward transmembrane current per unit volume is, in accordance with the conservation law (Eq. 4),

$$i_m = \nabla \cdot D_i\nabla\phi_i = -\nabla \cdot D_e\nabla\phi_e . \tag{6}$$

The transmembrane potential is defined in H as

$$v_m = \phi_i - \phi_e . \tag{7}$$

The terms $D_i\nabla\phi_e$ and $-D_i\nabla\phi_e$ can be added to Eq. 3 and, by using Eq. 7 and recalling that $D = D_i + D_e$, we get for the total current density

$$\mathbf{J} = -D_i\nabla v_m - D\nabla\phi_e = \mathbf{J}^i - D\nabla\phi_e . \tag{8}$$

Here $\mathbf{J}^i$ was substituted for $-D_i\nabla v_m$; this term has a dimension of a current dipole moment per unit volume and it is called an *impressed current density* [9]. The impressed current density is driven by the electrochemical generators in cardiac cells, while the term $-D\nabla\phi_e$ represents passive return currents in the tissue. From the condition that the divergence of $\mathbf{J}$ must vanish, or alternatively, by substitutions from Eq. 7 into Eq. 6, we can obtain a fundamental partial differential equation in ϕ_e, with a source term that involves the gradient of the transmembrane potential v_m (c.f. Geselowitz and Miller [7] Eqs. (4) and (7); Plonsey and Barr [10] Eq. (7))

$$\nabla \cdot D\nabla\phi_e = -\nabla \cdot D_i\nabla v_m = \nabla \cdot \mathbf{J}^i . \tag{9}$$

Thus, the distribution of the interstitial potential, ϕ_e, is related by Eq. 9 to the current sources. Eq. 9 suggests that H can be regarded as a composite medium characterized by the bulk conductivity tensor D, in which there is a distributed impressed current density (a current dipole moment per unit volume), defined by the term $\mathbf{J}^i = -D_i\nabla v_m$; the divergence of the latter is the impressed scalar current per unit volume [9].

From the cable theory [11] we have

$$i_m = \chi[C_m \frac{\partial v_m}{\partial t} + I_{ion} - I_{app}] \tag{10}$$

where χ is the membrane surface area per unit volume of the tissue, C_m is the membrane capacitance per unit area of the membrane surface, I_{ion} is the ionic current per unit area of the membrane surface, and I_{app} represents an applied current stimulus to start the activation. By combining Eqs. 6 and 10 and by defining

$$c_m = \chi C_m, \quad i_{ion} = \chi I_{ion}, \quad i_{app} = \chi I_{app},$$

we get an equation that relates the spatial distribution of intracellular potential and the membrane dynamics:

$$c_m \frac{\partial v_m}{\partial t} + i_{ion} - i_{app} = \nabla \cdot D_i \nabla \phi_i \quad \text{in } H. \tag{11}$$

By substituting $\phi_i = v_m + \phi_e$, we can rewrite Eq. 11 in terms of v_m and ϕ_e:

$$c_m \frac{\partial v_m}{\partial t} - \nabla \cdot D_i \nabla v_m + i_{ion}(v_m) = \nabla \cdot D_i \nabla \phi_e + i_{app} \quad \text{in } H. \tag{12}$$

In this form, we have in H a system composed of a nonlinear parabolic equation (Eq. 12) in v_m, coupled with an elliptic equation (Eq. 9) in ϕ_e.

Under the case of equal anisotropy ratio [10], $D_e = kD_i$, $\phi_e = -v_m/(k+1)$, and Eq. 12 becomes

$$c_m \frac{\partial v_m}{\partial t} = \frac{k}{k+1} \nabla \cdot D_i \nabla v_m - i_{ion}(v_m) + i_{app}, \tag{13}$$

while in B we have an elliptic equation (Eq. 5) in ϕ_o.

2.3 Boundary Conditions

Let the closed surface S_H be a boundary separating bidomain region H and surrounding volume conductor B, and let the closed surface S_B bound region B; $\mathbf{n}$ will denote the unit outward normal to S_H and S_B. Since the potential must be continuous at each boundary and the current must be continuous across each boundary,

$$\phi_o = \phi_e, \quad \mathbf{n} \cdot \sigma_o \nabla \phi_o = \mathbf{n} \cdot (D \nabla \phi_e + D_i \nabla v_m) \quad \text{on } S_H \tag{14}$$

$$\mathbf{n} \cdot \sigma_o \nabla \phi_o = 0 \quad \text{on } S_B. \tag{15}$$

The bidomain system in H and the passive volume conductor B are connected via transmission condition on the boundary S_H (Eq. 14). Since the sources in H are related to the presence of intracellular medium, which is absent in B, we may assume that the vector $D_i \nabla v_m$ in Eq. 14 is tangent to the surface S_H; this becomes an additional boundary condition:

$$\mathbf{n} \cdot D_i \nabla v_m = 0 \text{ on } S_H. \tag{16}$$

The same argument can be made for the vector $D_i \nabla \phi_i$

$$\mathbf{n} \cdot D_i \nabla \phi_i = 0 \text{ on } S_H. \tag{17}$$

The conditions 16 and 17 are analogous to the sealed-end condition in the one-dimensional cable model.

2.4 Extracardiac Fields

As presented above, the extracardiac potential ϕ_o can be solved everywhere in B according to Eq. 5 and the boundary conditions 14 and 15. The external magnetic field $\mathbf{B}(\mathbf{r})$ due to the total current density $\mathbf{J}$ from Eq. 3 can in turn be evaluated from the Biot-Savart law.

3 Solution of the Bidomain Equations

3.1 Dalhousie Propagation Model

Our propagation model was developed at Dalhousie University to simulate the electrical excitation wavefronts in two- and three-dimensional arrays of excitable cells [4]. Besides the anisotropic bidomain theory, the model comprises features from the cellular automata theory. To develop a model for simulating propagated excitation in large and complex cardiac network structure, the bisyncytium was tessellated into n subregions ($n \sim 10^6$). Each subregion is characterized by two static parameters: a cell type and a principal fiber direction a. Associated with each cell is a distinct set of electrophysiological parameters. It is assumed that the cell membrane has a voltage threshold v_{th}. Electrotonic interaction of the model's excitable elements is governed by the parabolic equation 13.

Formally, the model can be defined as a cellular automaton consisting of n interconnected finite state machines. The time domain is discretized into a set of time instants, $t_{k+1} = t_k + \delta t$, where δt is the discrete time step. Each cell is assigned its own space in the computer memory, where both static and dynamic information are stored. The static information specifies the cell type and the local fiber direction a (in terms of the angles Φ, Θ in the globally defined polar coordinate system). The cell's dynamic information consists of two components: the *macro-state* and the *micro-state*. Each cell can be in one of the four macro-states, which correspond to well-known distinct phases of the action potential: 1) the resting state, 2) the excitatory state, 3) the absolute refractory state, 4) the relative refractory state. There are 16 possible macro-state transitions between the four states, but physiological constraints reduce possible transitions to eleven. The states and the transitions are described in detail elsewhere [4,5].

3.2 Equal Anisotropy Ratio

The membrane potential $v_m(t+1)$ is solved from discretized Eq. 13 by explicit difference method for $v_m(t)$ [4,13]. Presently, the ionic current density i_{ion} in Eq. 13 includes only the inward rectifier i_{K1} [14]. The suprathreshold behavior of the elements depends only on time, the recovery interval and the cell type; it is largely determined by the state-transition rules of the cellular automaton [4,5].

The model has been previously tested in simulating the propagation in two- and three-dimensional arrays of cells [6,12], and also in a realistic geometry model of the human ventricles for simulating potential maps and magnetic field distributions of normal ventricular depolarization (Horáček et al., this volume).

3.3   General Anisotropy Ratio

In a general case, we have to solve the parabolic Eq. 12 and the elliptic Eq. 9, with the appropriate boundary conditions 14 and 16. The solution becomes computationally tedious, but can be achieved with utilizing the sparse nature of the discretized problem. For example, Roth [15] and Henriquez et al. [16] solved the elliptic equation 9 using an iterative method, and then substituted the resulting ϕ_e to Eq. 12.

The bidomain equations are solvable also in the context of Dalhousie hybrid model. If we rewrite Eq. 4 as $\nabla \cdot (D_i \nabla v_m + D \nabla \phi_e) = 0$, Eq. 12 becomes

$$c_m \frac{\partial v_m}{\partial t} = i_{\text{app}} - i_{\text{ion}}(v_m) - \nabla \cdot D_e \nabla \phi_e , \tag{18}$$

which needs to be solved simultaneously with Eq. 9:

$$\nabla \cdot D \nabla \phi_e = -\nabla \cdot D_i \nabla v_m . \tag{19}$$

1. Initially, $v_m(t = 0) = v_r$ in all cells, and selecting $\phi_i = 0$, $\phi_e(t = 0) = -v_r$.
2. When an external stimulus is applied at time t_k, solve $v_m(t_{k+1})$ as a function of $\phi_e(t_k)$, applying the explicit forward method to parabolic Eq. 18.
3. Substitute the resulting $v_m(t_{k+1})$ to the elliptic Eq. 19, and solve the distribution of $\phi_e(t_{k+1})$.
4. Switch to the next time point and repeat the previous two steps.

The fortran-language implementation was run on an IBM RS/6000 SP supercomputer at the CSC - Scientific Computing Ltd (Espoo, Finland; http://www.csc.fi). In solving the parabolic Eq. 18, we utilized the parallelized sparse system solvers of the ESSL library (http://www.rs6000.ibm.com/resource/aix_resource/sp_books/essl/).

4   Simulations

We performed computer simulations in an array of $100 \times 100 \times 10$ cells with the spacing of $h = 0.2$ mm. Initial stimulus was delivered at the center of the array and the excitation was propagated for 20 ms. Figure 1 displays the first test simulations for excitation isochrones (i.e., the times when v_m at each cell exceeds the threshold to trigger an action potential) for two sets of conductivities:

- For equal anisotropy ratio, Eq. 13, $\sigma_l^{i,e} = 2.5$ mS/cm, $\sigma_t^{i,e} = 0.6$ mS/cm.
- For unequal anisotropy ratio, Eqs. 18 and 19, $\sigma_l^i = 3$ mS/cm, $\sigma_t^i = 0.315$ mS/cm, $\sigma_l^e = 2$ mS/cm, $\sigma_t^e = 1.351$ mS/cm (according to [16] and [17]).
- Other parameters: $\delta t = 0.01$ ms, $C_m = 1.0$ μF/cm^2, $\chi = 2000$.

In the equal anisotropy ratio case, the axial and transversal propagation velocities were, respectively, about 1.0 and 0.5 mm/ms. The propagation ellipsoid for the general anisotropy showed a slightly 'slimmer' shape, the axial propagation velocity was about the same but the transversal propagation was slightly slower than in the equal anisotropy case.

a)   b)

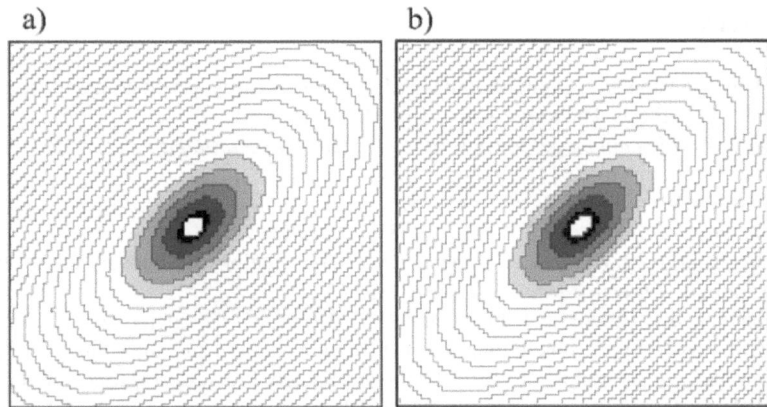

Fig. 1. Simulated isochrones for a) equal anisotropy ratio, and for b) unequal anisotropy ratio. The simulation parameter values are given in the text.

5   Discussion

In this study, the viewpoint is macroscopic, and each excitable element actually represents a large number ($\sim$1000) of myocardial cells. We used a fixed shape for the action potential above the threshold value, but the shape and duration can easily be altered to match experimentally measured action potentials or action potentials simulated with one- or two-dimensional cellular-scale models based on Luo-Rudy-type differential equations [14].

Previous studies of general anisotropy ratios (e.g. [15], [16]) were involving detailed characteristics of the ionic channels in fairly small blocks of excitable cells ($h \sim 100\mu m$). Such approach may not be easily extendable to a macroscopic view required in simulations of body surface maps. Our hybrid approach can in turn accommodate different grid sizes when special care is paid in defining the model parameters and difference formula [13].

The isochrones in our first simulations with general anisotropy ratios have elliptical shapes, and the estimated average propagation velocities are in fairly good agreement with the square-root relation $\vartheta_\ell/\vartheta_t = \sqrt{\sigma_\ell^i/\sigma_t^i}$ [18,19]. Moreover, the velocities are in agreement with the velocities estimated from in vitro experimental data [20].

Our model allows simulations of propagated excitation in large and complex anatomical structures, such as the ventricles, by assuming equal anisotropy ratio and bypassing accurate modelling of membrane ionic processes during the cardiac action potential. More general anisotropies can also be taken into account by increasing the computational demands (intercoupled elliptic and parabolic PDE). Still, more detailed simulations are required to study the effect of different anisotropy ratios, especially on body surface maps, and to validate the assumptions for the whole-heart simulations.

References

1. H.J. Ritsema van Eck, "Digital-computer simulation of cardiac excitation and repolarization in man". PhD thesis, Dalhousie University, Halifax, Canada, 1972.
2. L. Tung. *A bidomain model for describing ischemic myocardial d-c potentials*. PhD thesis, Massachusetts Institute of Technology, 1978.
3. W.T. Miller III and D.B. Geselowitz. Simulation studies of the electrocardiogram: I. The normal heart. *Circ Res*, 43: 301–315, 1978.
4. L.J. Leon and B.M. Horáček. Computer model of excitation and recovery in the anisotropic myocardium. *J Electrocardiol*, 24: 1–41, 1991.
5. J. Nenonen, J.A. Edens, L.J. Leon, and B.M. Horáček. Computer model of propagated excitation in the anisotropic human heart: I. Implementation and algorithms. In *Computers in Cardiology*, pages 545–548, IEEE Computer Society Press, Los Alamitos, CA, 1992.
6. B.M. Horáček, J. Nenonen, J.A. Edens, and L.J. Leon. A hybrid computer model of propagated excitation in the anisotropic human ventricular myocardium. In: *Biomedical and Life Physics*, D.N. Ghista, ed. (Viewer Verlag, Wiesbaden, 1996), pp. 181–190.
7. D.B. Geselowitz and W.T. Miller III. A bidomain model for anisotropic cardiac muscle. *Ann. Biomed. Eng.*, 11: 191–206, 1983.
8. P. Colli Franzone, L. Guerri, and S. Tentoni. Mathematical modelling of the excitation process in myocardial tissue: influence of fiber rotation on wavefront propagation and potential field. *Math. Biosci.*, 101: 155–235, 1990.
9. R. Plonsey. *Bioelectric Phenomena*. McGraw-Hill, New York, 1969.
10. R. Plonsey and R.C. Barr. Current flow patterns in two-dimensional anisotropic bisyncytia with normal and extreme conductivities. *Biophys J*, 45: 557–571, 1984.
11. J.J.B. Jack, D. Noble, and R.W. Tsien. *Electric Current Flow in Excitable Cells*. Clarendon Press, Oxford, 1975.
12. R. Hren, J. Nenonen, and B.M. Horacek, "Simulated epicardial potential maps during paced activation reflect myocardial fibrous structure". *Ann Biomed Eng* 26: 1022–1035, 1998.
13. K. Simelius, J. Nenonen, and B.M. Horáček. Bidomain simulations of cardiac activation with large elements. *Submitted.*
14. C.H. Luo and Y. Rudy. A dynamic model of the cardiac ventricular action potential I. Simulations of ionic currents and concentration changes. *Circ. Res.*, 74: 1071–1096, 1994.
15. B. Roth. Action potential propagation in a thick strand of cardiac muscle. *Circ. Res.*, 68: 162–173, 1991.
16. C.S. Henriquez, A.L. Muzikant, and C.K. Smoak. Anisotropy, fiber curvature, and bath loading effects on activation in thin and thick cardiac tissue preparations: Simulations in a three-dimensional bidomain model. *J. Cardiovasc. Electrophys.*, 7: 424–444, 1996.
17. B.J. Roth. Electrical conductivity values used with the bidomain model of cardiac tissue. *IEEE Trans. Biomed. Eng.*, 44: 326–328, 1997.
18. R.M. Gulrajani. Models of the electrical activity of the heart and computer simulation of the electrocardiogram. *CRC Crit Rev Biomed Eng* 16: 1–61, 1988.
19. A. Muler, and V. Markin. Electrical properties of anisotropic nerve-muscle bisyncytia – III. Steady form of the excitation front. *Biofizika* 22: 671–675, 1977.
20. D. Durrer, R.Th. van Dam, G.E. Freud, M.J. Janse, F.J. Mejler, and R.C. Artzbaecher. Total excitation of the isolated human heart. *Circulation* 41: 899–912, 1970.

Imaging of Electrical Function within the Human Atrium and Ventricle from Paced ECG Mapping Data

Bernhard Tilg[1], Robert Modre[1], Gerald Fischer[1,2], Friedrich Hanser[1], Bernd Messnarz[1], and Franz Xaver Roithinger[2]

[1] Graz University of Technology, Krenngasse 37, 8010 Graz, Austria,
bernhard.tilg@tugraz.at,
http://www-db.tu-graz.ac.at/start.htm
[2] Department of Cardiology, University Hospital Innsbruck,
Anichstrasse 35, 6020 Innsbruck, Austria

Abstract. Activation time (AT) imaging from electrocardiographic mapping data is under development becoming feasible for clinical applications. In this study the AT imaging approach is applied to data of the human atria and ventricles in four patients. The reconstructed atrial AT pattern on the endo- and epicardium for paced rhythm data was compared with the CARTO® map. The geometrical error between the modelled right atrial (RA) target chamber and the anatomical CARTO® map was between 4 and 7mm. With regard to the localization error we compared the locations of the first (endocardial) breakthroughs determined from the reconstructed AT map and from the CARTO® map within RA. This localization error was identified to be within 6 and 13mm.

1 Introduction

Combined magnetic resonance imaging (MRI) of the torso anatomy and electrocardiographic (ECG) mapping enables noninvasive imaging of the electrical function in the human heart [1,2,3,4,5]. Beside the imaging of cardiac movement, perfusion and metabolism, the reconstruction of electrical function will have a significant clinical impact.

The primary source in the cardiac muscle is the spatiotemporal transmembrane potential φ_m distribution. For depolarization, the assumption of electrical isotropy in the myocardium yields reasonable results [6,7]. Because of the unknown individual fiber orientation this hypothesis is considered in the *uniform dipole layer theory* based source model formulation. Herewith, the forward and inverse formulation can be reduced to a two-dimensional field and scalar potential problem. In general, the boundary element method is applied for this kind of problem [6].

In the inverse problem parameters describing features of φ_m or the epicardial (more precisely the pericardial) potential are estimated [1,2,4,8,5]. The epicardial

T. Katila et al. (Eds.): FIMH 2001, LNCS 2230, pp. 148–155, 2001.

potential as well as the potential on all other conductivity interfaces are related to φ_m by a Fredholm integral equation of 2nd order [6,7]. The most established inverse formulations are the imaging of the *activation time* (AT) map on the entire surface of the ventricle or the atrium (employing the uniform dipole layer or transmembrane potential source model formulation) and of the epicardial potential pattern (by solving the so-called *epicardial potential problem*) [1,2,9,4,8].

In clinical electrocardiology arrhythmias, in particular within the human atrium and their therapeutic treatment, play a major role [10]. In clinical practise, the localization of the origin of arrhythmias is currently achieved by traditional catheter techniques and by recently introduced catheter mapping techniques, e.g., by CARTO® (Biosense Webster Inc., A Johnson&Johnson company) [11]. These methods have limitations, e.g., they do not allow acquiring a single beat activation map and are to some extent time consuming. The single beat AT imaging approach would provide this information fully noninvasive and - at least theoretically - immediately after the ECG recording. From a clinical point of view this might have several advantages. The AT imaging methods permit the reconstruction of single focal, multiple focal, and more distributed activation patterns. Furthermore, these methods can distinguish between areas with early and late activation. Potential clinical applications of the ECG inverse problem are noninvasive imaging of atrial and ventricular ectopic as well as pre-excited activation.

In this study we investigated the applicability of the AT imaging method in four patients who underwent an electrophysiological (EP) study in the catheter laboratory. We focused on paced atrial and ventricular activation sequences.

2   Methods

Prior to the treatment in the catheter laboratory individual anatomical data were obtained by MRI using a Magnetom-Vision-Plus 1.5 Tesla scanner. Atrial and ventricular geometry was recorded in CINE-mode during breath-hold (expiration, 21×7 oblique short axis scans, 4 and 6mm spacing). The lungs and the torso shape were recorded in T1-FLASH-mode during breath-hold (expiration, 40 axial scans, 10mm spacing). 12 markers (vitamin E capsules, 7 anatomical landmarks on the anterior and lateral chest wall, 5 electrode positions on the patient's back) were used to couple the electrode positions and the reference points to the MRI frame. From this data set a boundary element volume conductor model was built up. Such a model is depicted in Fig. 1 from an anterior left lateral view for a 21-year old male patient suffering from the Wolff-Parkinson-White(WPW)-syndrome.

The patients were then moved to the catheter laboratory and ECG mapping data were recorded during and after the EP study. ECG mapping data were collected in 62-channels by the Mark-8 system (Biosemi V.O.F., Amsterdam, The Netherlands). A Wilson terminal defined the reference potential. The sampling rate was 2048 Hz. Signals were bandpass filtered with a lower and upper edge frequency of 0.3 Hz and 400 Hz, respectively. The AC-resolution of the system is

500 nV/bit (16 bit per channel). Radiotransparent carbon electrodes were used in order to allow simultaneous X-ray examination.

The position of the electrodes on the anterior and lateral chest wall was digitized by the Fastrak® system (Polhemus Inc., Colchester, Vermont). Additionally, the positions of the 7 anterior and lateral landmarks were digitized in order to allow coordinate transformation to the MRI frame. The locations of the 5 upper posterior electrodes were identical with the position of the 5 posterior MRI markers.

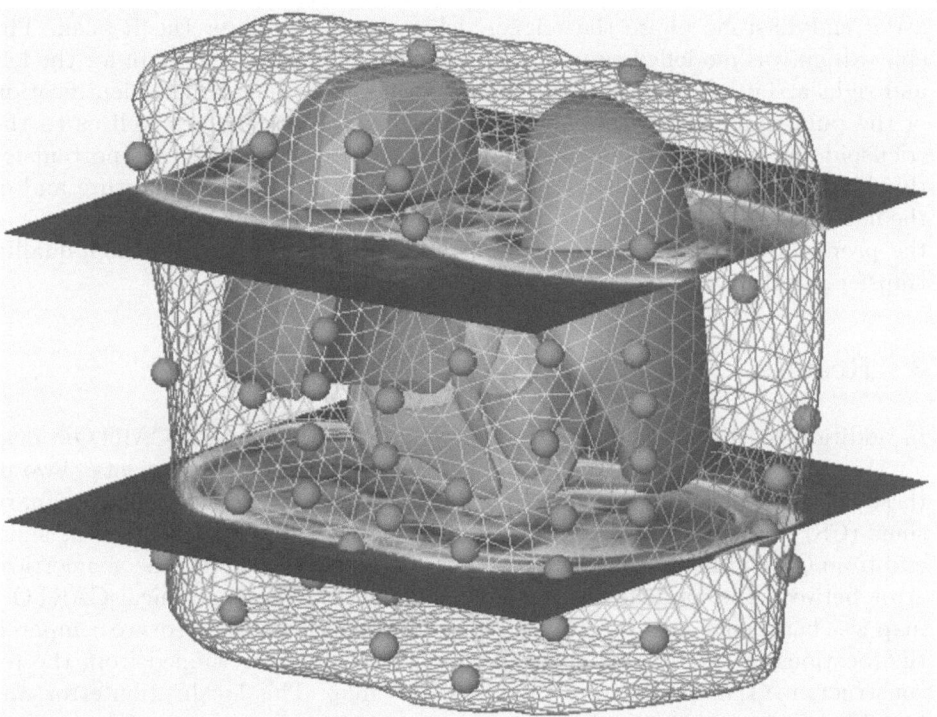

Fig. 1. Volume conductor model of a 21-year old male patient suffering from the WPW-syndrome. From the patient axial MRI scans for modelling the chest and the right and left lung, and ECG-gated short axis scans through the cardiac muscle for modelling the atrium (600ms) and the ventricle (0ms) were acquired. For this patient 45 electrodes (spheres) were considered for reconstructing the atrial and ventricular AT map. The ventricular and atrial surface model consisted of 616 and 674 nodal points (= unknowns), respectively. The Wilson terminal was considered as reference. The electrode and reference locations were acquired with the Fastrak® system in the catheter laboratory.

The ECG raw data were pre-processed by baseline correction, but no additional filtering was applied [12]. The transfer matrix was calculated applying the boundary element method with linear triangular elements considering the Wilson terminal [6]. The AT map was determined from single beat ECG mapping data applying an iterative linear inverse approach. Details on this inverse approach and on the AT imaging approach in general, can be found elsewhere [1,2,4].

Because of the complex anatomy of the human atrium there are several aspects in the evaluation of a "good" atrial surface model. Specific care has to be taken on the MRI protocol in obtaining scans with a high gray-value contrast. The atrial surface model shown in Fig. 2 and 3 was obtained from short-axis scans with 4mm slice thickness in a CINE-mode during breath-hold. For the atrial end-diastolic phase the trigger delay was 600ms after the R-peak. The epicardium was modelled assuming a uniform wall thickness of 4mm for the left and right atrial free wall. Specific attention has to be paid to the identification of the pulmonary veins, the vena cava inferior and superior as well as to the tricuspid and mitral annulus. The modeling of these structures is important for this kind of inverse formulation. Because of the sophisticated curvature and of the narrowness of the individual endo- and epicardial boundary element surfaces the proper meshing is of utmost importance in order to obtain a high-quality transfer matrix.

3   Results

In addition to the 62-channel ECG mapping and MRI data a CARTO® map for the right atrium (RA) was available from each of the four patients. Two of these maps were acquired during sinus rhythm, the other ones during a coronary sinus (CS) pacing protocol. AT imaging was performed from single beat sinus and from CS and high right atrium (HRA) paced rhythm data. The geometrical error between the modelled RA target chamber and the anatomical CARTO® map was between 4 and 7mm. With regard to the localization error we compared the locations of the first (endocardial) breakthroughs determined from the reconstructed AT map and from the CARTO® map. This localization error was identified to be within 6 and 13mm.

In order to give an example of the localization accuracy, two different atrial AT map reconstructions achieved from the 21-year old male patient's data set are shown in Fig. 2 and Fig 3. AT imaging was performed for HRA and CS pacing. Reconstruction was done from single beat data. For this localization protocol the ECG mapping data and the corresponding CARTO® maps were acquired at the end of the EP study, after successful ablation of the accessory pathway.

Firstly, a pacing catheter was placed in the HRA of RA, creating a virtual triangle with RAA and VCS. The reconstructed AT map is depicted in Fig. 2. It can be seen clearly, that the origin of this paced propagation wave is properly found. In this case, however, only an anatomical marker was available for comparison. Secondly, the pacing catheter was moved to the CS-Ostium location and the stimuli protocol was continued. Again, the propagation pattern was reconstructed very well from the stimulated target P wave as can be seen in Fig. 3.

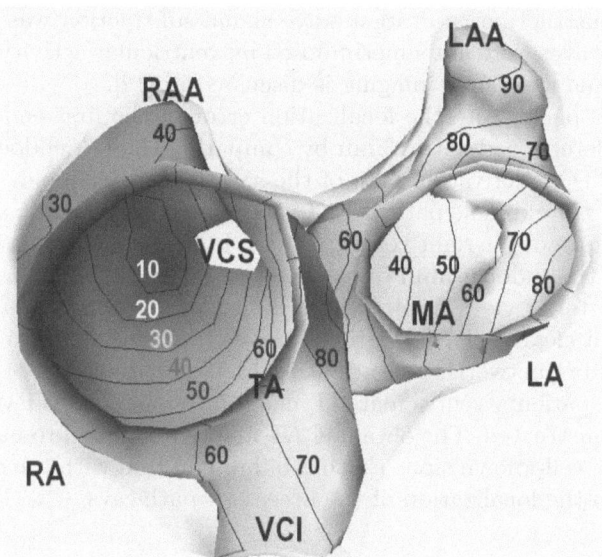

Fig. 2. Endocardial activation time map in ms for the HRA pacing protocol seen from a caudal oblique view. Isochrones are depicted in steps of 10ms. The following abbreviations are used: Right atrium (RA), left atrium (LA), right atrial appendage (RAA), left atrial appendage (LAA), vena cava inferior (VCI), vena cava superior (VCS), tricuspid annulus (TA), mitral annulus (MA)

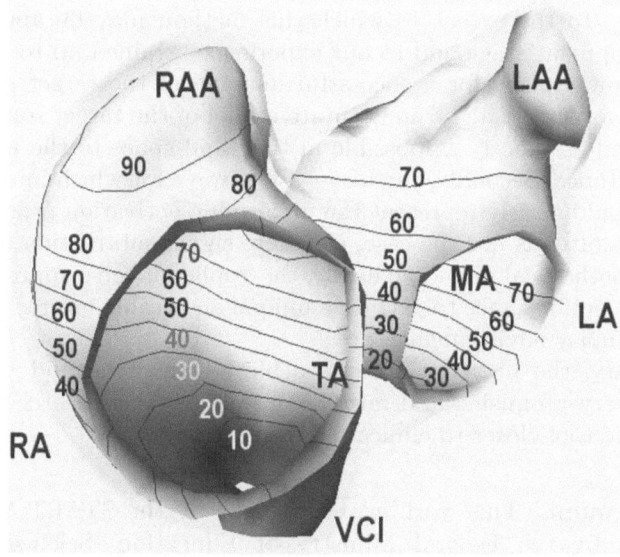

Fig. 3. Endocardial activation time map in ms for the CS-Ostium pacing protocol seen from a caudal right lateral oblique view. Isochrones are depicted in steps of 10ms. Abbreviations as in Fig. 2.

For both reconstructions no target wave signal-subtraction was necessary. The stimulated P waves were not superimposed by ventricular activity. The relevance of this technique for source imaging is discussed in [12].

For the CS pacing site the localization error of the first endocardial breakthrough was determined with 13mm by comparing the RA endocardial AT map with the CARTO® activation map of the same target chamber.

In this 21-year old male patient ECG mapping data were also acquired during pacing of the apex of the right ventricle (RV). In Fig. 4 the reconstructed AT map is depicted on the endocardium (upper panel) and epicardium (lower panel) from an anterior posterior view. Again, reconstruction was done from single beat data. As can be seen clearly, the activation spreads from the RV pacing site through the Purkinje fibre network to the right and left ventricular (LV) free wall.

In all four patients ventricular AT maps for sinus and WPW-sinus rhythm data were reconstructed. The obtained AT maps were found to be in good agreement with the well-known sinus rhythm in humans and with the clinical findings with regard to the localization of the accessory pathways.

4 Discussion

We demonstrated that AT imaging within the human atrium and ventricle from paced and sinus rhythm ECG mapping data is feasible under clinical conditions. Of course, the imaging of spontaneous rhythms, like the onset of flutter or spontaneous foci from the pulmonary veins, will be another important milestone in the development and clinical establishment of this novel diagnostic imaging technique. To the extent to which this method may be applicable at the present development stage and to our experience attained up to now, there are some important aspects for a successful imaging of the target activation pattern. Firstly, not surprisingly, an accurate model of the target source-containing surface coupled as exactly as possible in time and space to the ECG data is of utmost importance. Secondly, the target ECG wave for which imaging has to be performed should clearly represent the underlying activation process. In clinical situations this often is not the case, therefore signal-subtraction techniques will have a huge methodical impact. Thirdly, the applied inverse approach must have the numerical performance to extract a unique and stable inverse solution in the presence of a noisy environment.

In summary, the presented results achieved on atrial and ventricular AT imaging are very promising and raise hope that further research will bring this new diagnostic tool closer to clinical applications.

Acknowledgment. This work was supported by the START Y144-INF program funded by the Federal Ministry of Education, Science and Culture (BmBWK) in collaboration with the Austrian Science Fund (FWF), Vienna, Austria. We are indebted to Maria Abou-Harb for her technical assistance in the catheter laboratory and to Michael Schocke for his help in acquiring MRI data.

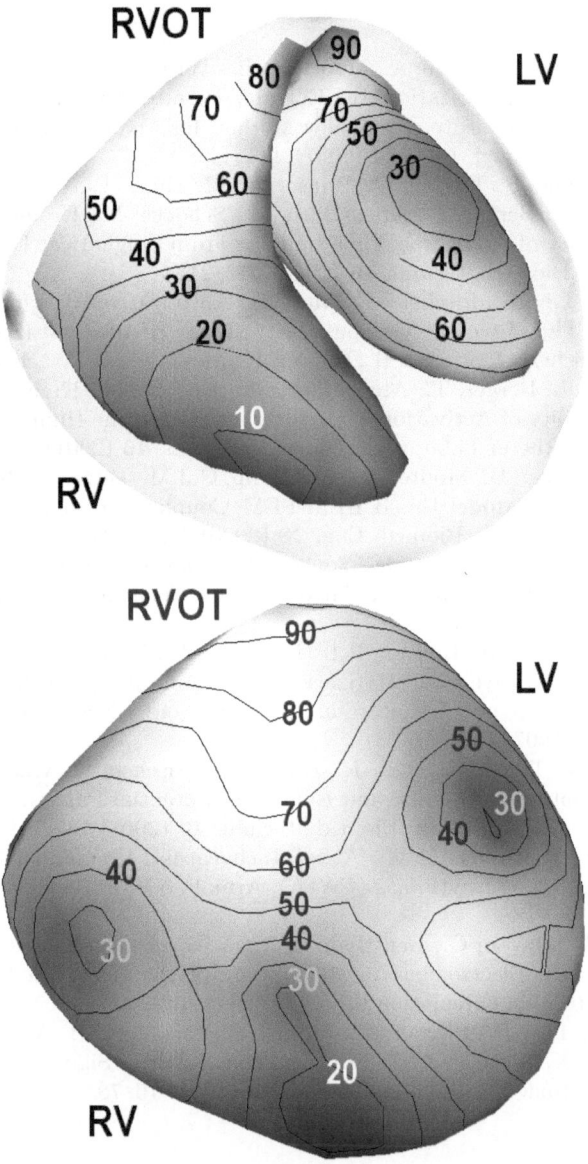

Fig. 4. Endo- (upper panel) and epicardial (lower panel) activation time map in ms for the RV pacing protocol seen from an anterior posterior view. Isochrones are depicted in steps of 10ms. The following abbreviations are used: Right ventricle (RV), left ventricle (LV), right ventricular outflow tract (RVOT)

References

1. Cuppen, J., van Oosterom, A.: Model Studies With Inversely Calculated Isochrones of Ventricular Depolarization. IEEE Trans. Biomed. Eng. **78** (1982) 315–333
2. Huiskamp, G., Greensite, F.: A new Method for Myocardial Activation Imaging. IEEE Trans. Biomed. Eng. **44** (1997) 433–446
3. Modre, R., Tilg, B., Fischer, G., Hanser, F., Messnarz, B., Wach, P., Pachinger, O., Hintringer, F., Berger, T., Abou-Harb, M., Schocke, M., Kremser, C., Roithinger, F.X.: Stability of Activation Time Imaging From Single Beat Data Under Clinical Conditions. Biomed. Technik **46** (2001) 213–215
4. Modre, R., Tilg, B., Fischer, G., Wach, P.: An Iterative Algorithm for Myocardial Activation Time Imaging. Comput. Meth. Prog. Biomed. **64** (2001) 1–7
5. Tilg, B., Fischer, G., Modre, R., Hanser, F., Messnarz, B., Wach, P., Pachinger, O., Hintringer, F., Berger, T., Abou-Harb, M., Schocke, M., Kremser, C., Roithinger, F.X.: Feasibility of Activation Time Imaging Within the Human Atria and Ventricles in the Catheter Laboratory. Biomed. Technik **46** (2001) 223–225
6. Fischer, G., Tilg., B., Modre., R., Huiskamp, G.J.M., Fetzer, J., Rucker, W., Wach, P.: A Bidomain Model Based BEM-FEM Coupling Formulation for Anisotropic Cardiac Tissue. Ann. Biomed. Eng. **28** (2000) 1229–1243
7. Yamashita, Y., Geselowitz, D.: Sourcefield Relationships for Cardiac Generators on the Heart Surface Based on Their Transfer Coefficients. IEEE Trans. Biomed. Eng. **632** (1985) 964–970
8. Oster, H.S., Taccardi, B., Lux, R.L., Ershler, P.R., Rudy, Y.: Electrocardiographic Imaging. Noninvasive Characterization of Intramural Myocardial Activation From Inversely Reconstructed Epicardial Potentials and Electrograms. Circulation **97** (1998) 1496–1507
9. Messnarz, B., Tilg, B., Modre, R., Hanser, F., Fischer, G., Wach, P.: Comparison of Transmembrane Potential and Epicardial Potential Patterns Reconstructed by a Linear Inverse Approach. Biomed. Technik **46** (2001) 147–149
10. Lesh, M.D., Roithinger, F.X.: Atrial Tachycardia, In: Camm, A.J. Clinical Approaches to Tachyarrhythmias (CATA), Armok, NY, Futura Publishing Company Inc., 2000.
11. Gepstein, L., Hayam G., Ben-Haim, S.A.: A Novel Method for Non-fdluoroscopic Catheter-based Electroanatomical Mapping of the Heart: In Vitro and in Vivo Accuracy Results. Circulation **95** (1997) 1611–1622 1997
12. Hanser, F., Tilg, B., Fischer, G., Modre, R., Messnarz, B., Wach, P., Berger, T., Pachinger, O., Hintringer, F., Roithinger, F.X.: ECG Signal Subtraction for Cardiac Source Imaging. Biomed. Technik **46** (2001) 76–78

Author Index

Lecture Notes in Computer Science

For information about Vols. 1–2144
please contact your bookseller or Springer-Verlag

Vol. 2184: M. Tucci (Ed.), Multimedia Databases and Image Communication. Proceedings, 2001. X, 225 pages. 2001.

Vol. 2185: M. Gogolla, C. Kobryn (Eds.), «UML» 2001 – The Unified Modeling Language. Proceedings, 2001. XIV, 510 pages. 2001.

Vol. 2186: J. Bosch (Ed.), Generative and Component-Based Software Engineering. Proceedings, 2001. VIII, 177 pages. 2001.

Vol. 2187: U. Voges (Ed.), Computer Safety, Reliability and Security. Proceedings, 2001. XVI, 249 pages. 2001.

Vol. 2188: F. Bomarius, S. Komi-Sirviö (Eds.), Product Focused Software Process Improvement. Proceedings, 2001. XI, 382 pages. 2001.

Vol. 2189: F. Hoffmann, D.J. Hand, N. Adams, D. Fisher, G. Guimaraes (Eds.), Advances in Intelligent Data Analysis. Proceedings, 2001. XII, 384 pages. 2001.

Vol. 2190: A. de Antonio, R. Aylett, D. Ballin (Eds.), Intelligent Virtual Agents. Proceedings, 2001. VIII, 245 pages. 2001. (Subseries LNAI).

Vol. 2191: B. Radig, S. Florczyk (Eds.), Pattern Recognition. Proceedings, 2001. XVI, 452 pages. 2001.

Vol. 2192: A. Yonezawa, S. Matsuoka (Eds.), Metalevel Architectures and Separation of Crosscutting Concerns. Proceedings, 2001. XI, 283 pages. 2001.

Vol. 2193: F. Casati, D. Georgakopoulos, M.-C. Shan (Eds.), Technologies for E-Services. Proceedings, 2001. X, 213 pages. 2001.

Vol. 2194: A.K. Datta, T. Herman (Eds.), Self-Stabilizing Systems. Proceedings, 2001. VII, 229 pages. 2001.

Vol. 2195: H.-Y. Shum, M. Liao, S.-F. Chang (Eds.), Advances in Multimedia Information Processing – PCM 2001. Proceedings, 2001. XX, 1149 pages. 2001.

Vol. 2196: W. Taha (Ed.), Semantics, Applications, and Implementation of Program Generation. Proceedings, 2001. X, 219 pages. 2001.

Vol. 2197: O. Balet, G. Subsol, P. Torguet (Eds.), Virtual Storytelling. Proceedings, 2001. XI, 213 pages. 2001.

Vol. 2198: N. Zhong, Y. Yao, J. Liu, S. Ohsuga (Eds.), Web Intelligence: Research and Development. Proceedings, 2001. XVI, 615 pages. 2001. (Subseries LNAI).

Vol. 2199: J. Crespo, V. Maojo, F. Martin (Eds.), Medical Data Analysis. Proceedings, 2001. X, 311 pages. 2001.

Vol. 2200: G.I. Davida, Y. Frankel (Eds.), Information Security. Proceedings, 2001. XIII, 554 pages. 2001.

Vol. 2201: G.D. Abowd, B. Brumitt, S. Shafer (Eds.), Ubicomp 2001: Ubiquitous Computing. Proceedings, 2001. XIII, 372 pages. 2001.

Vol. 2202: A. Restivo, S. Ronchi Della Rocca, L. Roversi (Eds.), Theoretical Computer Science. Proceedings, 2001. XI, 440 pages. 2001.

Vol. 2204: A. Brandstädt, V.B. Le (Eds.), Graph-Theoretic Concepts in Computer Science. Proceedings, 2001. X, 329 pages. 2001.

Vol. 2205: D.R. Montello (Ed.), Spatial Information Theory. Proceedings, 2001. XIV, 503 pages. 2001.

Vol. 2206: B. Reusch (Ed.), Computational Intelligence. Proceedings, 2001. XVII, 1003 pages. 2001.

Vol. 2207: I.W. Marshall, S. Nettles, N. Wakamiya (Eds.), Active Networks. Proceedings, 2001. IX, 165 pages. 2001.

Vol. 2208: W.J. Niessen, M.A. Viergever (Eds.), Medical Image Computing and Computer-Assisted Intervention – MICCAI 2001. Proceedings, 2001. XXXV, 1446 pages. 2001.

Vol. 2209: W. Jonker (Ed.), Databases in Telecommunications II. Proceedings, 2001. VII, 179 pages. 2001.

Vol. 2210: Y. Liu, K. Tanaka, M. Iwata, T. Higuchi, M. Yasunaga (Eds.), Evolvable Systems: From Biology to Hardware. Proceedings, 2001. XI, 341 pages. 2001.

Vol. 2211: T.A. Henzinger, C.M. Kirsch (Eds.), Embedded Software. Proceedings, 2001. IX, 504 pages. 2001.

Vol. 2212: W. Lee, L. Mé, A. Wespi (Eds.), Recent Advances in Intrusion Detection. Proceedings, 2001. X, 205 pages. 2001.

Vol. 2213: M.J. van Sinderen, L.J.M. Nieuwenhuis (Eds.), Protocols for Multimedia Systems. Proceedings, 2001. XII, 239 pages. 2001.

Vol. 2214: O. Boldt, H. Jürgensen (Eds.), Automata Implementation. Proceedings, 1999. VIII, 183 pages. 2001.

Vol. 2215: N. Kobayashi, B.C. Pierce (Eds.), Theoretical Aspects of Computer Software. Proceedings, 2001. XV, 561 pages. 2001.

Vol. 2216: E.S. Al-Shaer, G. Pacifici (Eds.), Management of Multimedia on the Internet. Proceedings, 2001. XIV, 373 pages. 2001.

Vol. 2217: T. Gomi (Ed.), Evolutionary Robotics. Proceedings, 2001. XI, 139 pages. 2001.

Vol. 2218: R. Guerraoui (Ed.), Middleware 2001. Proceedings, 2001. XIII, 395 pages. 2001.

Vol. 2220: C. Johnson (Ed.), Interactive Systems. Proceedings, 2001. XII, 219 pages. 2001.

Vol. 2221: D.G. Feitelson, L. Rudolph (Eds.), Job Scheduling Strategies for Parallel Processing. Proceedings, 2001. VII, 207 pages. 2001.

Vol. 2224: H.S. Kunii, S. Jajodia, A. Sølvberg (Eds.), Conceptual Modeling – ER 2001. Proceedings, 2001. XIX, 614 pages. 2001.

Vol. 2225: N. Abe, R. Khardon, T. Zeugmann (Eds.), Algorithmic Learning Theory. Proceedings, 2001. XI, 379 pages. 2001. (Subseries LNAI).

Vol. 2229: S. Qing, T. Okamoto, J. Zhou (Eds.), Information and Communications Security. Proceedings, 2001. XIV, 504 pages. 2001.

Vol. 2230: T. Katila, I.E. Magnin, P. Clarysse, J. Montagnat, J. Nenonen (Eds.), Functional Imaging and Modeling of the Heart. Proceedings, 2001. XI, 158 pages. 2001.

Vol. 2232: L. Fiege, G. Mühl, U. Wilhelm (Eds.), Electronic Commerce. Proceedings, 2001. X, 233 pages. 2001.

Vol. 2233: J. Crowcroft, M. Hofmann (Eds.), Networked Group Communication. Proceedings, 2001. X, 205 pages. 2001.

Vol. 2239: T. Walsh (Ed.), Principles and Practice of Constraint Programming – CP 2001. Proceedings, 2001. XIV, 788 pages. 2001.

Vol. 2241: M. Jünger, D. Naddef (Eds.), Computational Combinatorial Optimization. IX, 305 pages. 2001.